Registered Nursing:

Tips & Tidbits

By

Lance Hansard

with

Richard Lamphier, RN.

DEDICATION

We dedicate this book to all past, present, and future nurses. We say thank you.

ACKNOWLEDGEMENTS

A special thanks to our family, friends, and coworkers that have made this book a reality.

CONTENTS

PREFACE

The day couldn't have been any worse: two doctors yelling, a boss with an attitude, three patient complaints, and a flux of overbearing family members. The ride home from work was filled with tears, and then the realization set in, "they didn't train me for this."

Being a nurse is a hard job. Regardless of the training that leads to certification as a Registered Nurse, there is always a deficit. Nothing can prepare nurses for the daily frustrations of the job. Nurse training programs are primarily aimed at creating effective and technically capable nurses. Nursing is stressful and handling that stress determines one's effectiveness as a nurse.

Registered Nursing: Tips & Tidbits acts like a mentor for nurses. The book is broken down into key areas for the purpose of helping nurses understand and deal with the fact that there is more to nursing than just the technical information taught in the classroom. The informal style allows readers to grasp key concepts. The book is designed to help nurses by giving specific examples, offering general tips that help make the job of nursing easier, and narratives by veteran nurses.

-Lance Hansard and Richard Lamphier, RN.

-1-

Being a Nurse

"Nursing is an art: and if it is to be made an art, it requires an exclusive devotion as hard a preparation, as any painter's or sculptor's work; for what is the having to do with dead canvas or dead marble, compared with having to do with the living body, the temple of God's spirit? It is one of the Fine Arts: I had almost said, the finest of Fine Arts."

-Florence Nightingale

Introduction

Becoming a nurse takes hard work, dedication, and determination. School offers the tools and the education to become a nurse, but when school is over and the job begins, are you really ready? Only time will tell. No matter how intensive the training is in a nursing school program, the education truly begins with your first job as a nurse, and the education comes in the form of on-the-job training.

The first day on the job can either be exciting, intimidating, or both. Sometimes, but not always, nurses feel overwhelmed on the first day on the job when they are officially no longer a student. Preceptors can only show new nurses so much; the rest becomes on-the-job training.

Every seasoned nurse has a story to share, and the longer nurses work in the field, the more stories they have. Every career has a starting point. Good, bad, or indifferent, people usually remember the first day on the job. The following story shares the memory of Richard Lamphier, a thirty-year veteran Registered Nurse, about his first day on the job working in a hospital.

Richard's First Day

I set my alarm clock to wake up early so I could make a fifty-mile commute to the inner-city teaching hospital where I so desperately wanted to work. At the time, I could not afford to live any closer, and public transportation was not an option. I remember getting dressed in my new scrubs. They were hospital-issued, white, and had the university patch sewn neatly on the right shoulder. I checked my chest in the mirror at least a dozen times to make sure my embroidered name was spelled correctly. I had spent at least an hour the night before pressing the wrinkles out of my uniform. Getting dressed was never so exciting because this time I did so as a Registered Nurse. Being a nursing student was behind me. My stomach felt a bit queasy as my nerves were trying to get the best of me. Shake it off, I kept telling myself. It's just a job. I must have repeated that phrase to myself a hundred times along with self-assuring comments like, "I can do this." I battled my nerves all morning. Getting ready seemed to take forever. I ate breakfast in a hurry, barely tasted my food, and had one thing on my mind: I can't be late.

I rushed out of the house, jumped into my car, fumbled with the keys, and finally managed to get the right key in the ignition. After cranking the Volkswagen Beetle that had faithfully served me all the way through nursing school, I pulled out of the driveway in plenty of time to get to work, prayed that my car wouldn't stall, and reassured myself that I was ready to save the world one patient at a time. Steadily making my way to the hospital that queasy feeling in my stomach was still nagging at me.

In the hospital orientation I received a parking garage map, and I looked it over several times as I navigated to the right parking lot. I read the name and floor of the designated nurse parking lot as I pulled up to the security gate. The security guard motioned me through after seeing my parking pass hanging from the rear view mirror. Pulling forward, I read the pass again because it said "nurse parking" on it. I was so excited to finally be there. I found an empty spot and pulled in. Digging around in a pile of papers that were sitting on the passenger seat I found my new stethoscope. I hung it around my neck, jumped out of the car, and headed toward the unit where I was to be working. I did it. Arriving promptly at 06:15 for my 07:00 shift, it felt like winning an award.

The night-shift nurses were nice when I arrived at the main nurses' station. Then the questions began: Is this your first day? Is this your first job as a nurse? How did they know? The assessment skills of these experienced nurses were impeccable. Will I ever be so observant? While standing around the nurses' station, one of the nurses spoke up and said, "You might want to take the price tag off your shiny new stethoscope." The crowd laughed.

I tried to hide my embarrassment, but it didn't work. My face had already blushed. I decided to just stand there quietly and wait on the charge nurse; I didn't want to bring any more attention to myself. The other day-shift nurses trickled in one by one. As each one arrived, I kept guessing if that nurse was going to be my preceptor. After what seemed to be an eternity, the charge nurse showed up just five minutes before the start of the shift. She wasted no time assigning room numbers and patients to each of the nurses at the station. She put my name next to the nurse named Debbie. I scribbled down my assignments on a notepad. When she had finished giving out our assignments, I noticed we had six patients assigned to us for the day. I thought the rules said there are supposed to be no more than four patients per nurse. Where's Debbie?

After everyone else had split up and departed the nurses' station, the night-shift nurse I was relieving was just standing there staring at me. Finally, she said, "Debbie will be here in a minute. Let's get started." I thrust my hand forward and introduced myself. Begrudgingly, the other nurse shook my hand. I could tell that she could not care less who I was. The nurse wasn't big on small talk and just started giving me reports on the patients. The nurse was talking so fast it was impossible for me to keep up. I decided rather hastily that note taking was going to be impossible at that point. So, I elected to just listen as we walked down the hall in front of my assigned patients' rooms. I asked her, "shouldn't we go in and check on the patients?" She said, "No, you can do that when Debbie gets here."

The nurse finished giving me the reports on four of the patients and didn't bother to ask me if I had any questions. Instead, she just turned and walked away. At this point, I was a bit confused. I raised my voice and asked, "What about the other two patients?" She continued down the hall and grumbled, "Not my patients, check the clipboard." Gradually the realization of what just happened set in, and a thought popped into my head, why did that nurse only have four patients last night and today I have six? A feeling of despair crept up on me as I trudged down the hall toward the nurses' station.

When I arrived at the station, there was no one there. I stared blankly at the charge nurse's clipboard that had the patient names written in one column and the room numbers written in the next column. I found the names of the last two patients assigned to me. I followed the lines to find out what nurse was caring for those two patients last night. When my eyes got to the column that had the nurses' names written in them I discovered that the name written in both of the boxes for these two patients was mine. They already changed the assignment board. Now what? Two patients and no report. My brain became frenzied, and then I had an idea: just check the charts. I don't know why I panicked. I guess my nerves were getting the best of me and it was only fifteen minutes into my shift.

I found the two corresponding charts sitting in the chart stand, pulled them out, and walked over to a chair that was at the nurses' desk to sit down. While flipping through the charts reading and searching for information about the patients, a voice suddenly boomed out, "Can't you hear the nurse call light?" Scared, shocked, and totally caught by surprise, I looked up and the charge nurse was standing on the other side of the desk looking down at me. Before answering her, the voice boomed again, "Where is your preceptor? The patient in room 502 says that she has called four times and no one has answered." My heart sank into the pit of my stomach. Not knowing what to do, I can't imagine what my face must have looked like at that moment. One of fear and confusion would be my guess, because the charge nurse took a minute and watched me squirm in my seat.

My mouth went dry while I was trying to answer, and I began to stutter a bit, "I…I don't know where she is. I … uh… I haven't seen her. The other nurse said she was running late and would be here in a minute."

"That just won't do. You have to make sure to answer the call lights." Her tone was very authoritative and made me feel small and insignificant. "Go check your patients. They are calling for a nurse. You are a nurse, aren't you?"

Without even answering her, I just got up and hurried down the hall. When I got to the patient's room she had her finger poised on the call button and she was rapidly pushing the button over and over. The call system was blinking and dinging at the head of her bed. I don't even know how to turn this damn thing off.

The patient yelled out, "You aren't Debbie, the night nurse said that Debbie was my nurse. Some man dressed in white shows up. I called for a nurse, who the hell are you?" I politely answered that I was her nurse and that Debbie would be here soon. I asked how I could help her. She snapped, "I need my pain medications. Can I get my pain medications? I asked for them 40 minutes ago." The voice stabbed at me across the room.

"Yes ma'am," I answered, "I will go and get them right now." I rushed out of the room and went to the chart holder to see exactly what pain medications she was asking for. I found the order in the chart and wrote down the exact medication and dose. This took me about five minutes. After going over to the medicine cart to get her pain medications, I realized that I needed the narcotic keys to open the cabinet.

The call system went off again. I turned around and saw that the light beside room 502 was blinking. It was Mrs. X again. I figured out how to work the intercom and asked how I could help her. She was yelling for her pain medications. I explained to her that I was getting them right now and that it would be just a few more minutes. By the tone in her voice, I don't think she believed me.

I asked the first nurse that went by, "Where are the keys for the narcotic cabinet?" A shrug of the shoulders and a blank stare was my answer. By this time I was getting mad at that stupid cart and was cursing it with every thought. A second nurse came by and I asked her the same question. She answered, "Ask your preceptor." Now I was full-blown mad. The thought of kicking the cart crossed my mind several times. Instead, I wandered the halls looking for a nurse who had the keys to no avail. I went back to the nurses' station just in time to answer the third call from Mrs. X.

"I see you figured out the call system," a voice said over my shoulder. I turned and looked. It was the charge nurse standing there glaring at me. I guess I was too focused on answering Mrs. X to hear her walk up behind me. She reached out with her hand and gave me the narcotic keys and said, "Make sure you give them back to me; that way the next nurse will know where to find them. The charge nurse should always have the narcotic keys." Her condescending voice grated at me. My heart sank. I had never felt so dumb in my whole life. In orientation, they emphasized that the charge nurse is responsible for the narcotic keys. After opening the cart, she snatched the keys back from me, turned, and walked away without a word. So, I pulled out the morphine, drew up 4 milligrams in a syringe and headed toward Mrs. X's room.

As I entered the room, Mrs. X's doctor was standing at the foot of her bed. The doctor had Mrs. X's chart in his hand and slammed it shut. He just stood there for a minute and began looking me over. I was standing there with a syringe in my hand confused and dazed. The doctor asked, "Is that Mrs. X's pain medications?"

"Yes sir," I answered.

His voice raised a few octaves as he explained to me that Mrs. X's pain medications were due at 06:30. By the time he was finished talking to me, he was very loud and I noticed a smile creep across Mrs. X's face as I just stood there being yelled at. He finished his rant with the question, "What took you so long?"

I felt small and humiliated. I didn't know how to answer or what to say. I had no excuse to offer. I didn't dare say that it was the night nurse's fault. It was my first day, and I was not about to get labeled as a tattletale. Mustering enough courage to apologize, I agreed with the doctor that there was no valid excuse. The doctor apparently had enough of berating me and he stormed out of the room. I was a bit shaken, but not deterred. Mrs. X was about to get her pain medications. It had taken me another fifteen minutes to get this medication ready, and there was another five-minute exchange with the doctor; I was not about to make her wait any longer. So, I swabbed the IV port, stabbed the needle in the line, and pushed the plunger with a lot of force and in a hurry.

Mrs. X started yelling, screaming, and kicking. "It burns, it burns! What did you do to me?" She started clawing at the IV line, and then the thought hit me. I didn't dilute the morphine. One might think that I would have been more sympathetic toward Mrs. X, but with how my morning was going this mistake was just one more thrown on the pile. I explained to her that it would pass in a minute and there was no need to worry. I don't think she believed me for a minute. I flushed the line several times to stop the burning, and I managed to keep Mrs. X from jerking her IV line out. The pain soon subsided but it was too late; Mrs. X now hated me.

Betty, the nursing assistant, called my name from the door. Using that as an excuse to escape the dagger-like eyes of Mrs. X, I left the room in a hurry. In the hallway, Betty told me that Mr. Y in room 505 needed me. In a few short strides I was at his room. I pushed the door open and a stench struck my nose. The smell was unbearable. I walked into the room and saw Mr. Y lying in the bed. The bed sheets right over his pelvic area were soaked with blood and urine. I couldn't believe the smell, and Mr. Y was just lying there calmly like nothing unusual was going on. After pulling the sheets back, Mr. Y said, "I think the hose fell out," in a calm voice. I began to feel a bit queasy.

"What did you do to him?" a voice squealed. I turned and looked. There was a young woman standing in the room with a terrified look on her face as she clasped her hands around her mouth. Wide-eyed, she stood mesmerized by the horrific sight of her father lying in a bloody mess.

"It's ok," I offered. "The catheter came out. Nothing to worry about," I said trying to be confident and reassuring.

"How can you say it is alright? Look at that. I am no doctor but that isn't right," she snapped. "How could you have let this happen to him?"

I didn't know how to answer those questions. I didn't do it, yet I was blamed for it. Instead of defending myself, I decided to retreat. "I'll be right back," I said as I left the room. "I will go get another Foley and something to clean him up with." When I got out into the hallway I remember taking a deep breath and fighting the urge to throw up. Heading back to the nurses' station, I ran into a nurse that I hadn't seen. "You must be Richard," she said. I hoped she was Debbie, my preceptor. After introductions, I found out that she was indeed Debbie. I tried to explain the mess in Mr. Y's room. She told me to get his chart, find his doctor's phone number, and call it. So, I did. But instead of reaching the doctor, I got the answering service, which told me that the office didn't open until nine o'clock. Then, they asked me if I would like to leave a message. I screamed into the phone, "I need to talk to the doctor now, this man is bleeding!" The doctor promptly called me back—ten minutes later. He gave me instructions on what to do until he got there. By the time I got to the supply room the idea of vomiting had passed. I got the supplies I needed, and after some searching, I found a technician to help me clean Mr. Y. I put the clots into a tray just like the doctor told me. I arranged the Foley supplies so that I would be ready when the doctor gave me the go ahead to reinsert the catheter—if needed.

The doctor said he would be there in twenty minutes. Instead, it took him thirty. Every five minutes, Mr. Y's daughter would stick her head in the door and ask me when the doctor was going to show up. Each time I answered, "He is on his way." Little did I know at the time, that same question would be asked every single day on the job. "When is the doctor going to show up?"

The rest of the day was a blur. I lost count of how many mistakes I had made that day. I remember finally getting to clock out and the long walk back to my car. I felt like a general who had just lost his army in a battle. I was the sole survivor of a war. I was alone and no one cared. I don't remember driving home, but I do remember how foggy my head felt as I pulled my car into the driveway. I turned the car off and just sat there for a while. There was only one thought that kept running through my head: they did not train me for this.

-Richard Lamphier, RN.

Connection

Richard's story illustrates how nursing school cannot prepare students for everything that a nurse may encounter while on the job. It takes time, experience, and practice to determine exactly what being a nurse really means. Each day is a new adventure and nurses should expect to be faced with situations that they may not be trained for. Embrace the challenge and keep in mind that all structures must begin with a foundation. Each day on the job builds that foundation. Using Richard's story as an example, he had a terrible first day, and things were not as he expected. However, thirty years later, Richard loves his job and still gets excited about going to work. Despite the rocky start, Richard realizes that that experience was all part of the process of building a solid foundation.

Processes

As with any process, mastering the practice of nursing will take time, and nurses shouldn't be surprised if it takes an entire career. In the beginning, the knowledge expected may be overwhelming. The nursing fundamentals book—no matter who the publisher—is a testament to this fact as it is well over one thousand pages of text packed with tremendous amounts of information that is covered in as little as ten weeks in some nursing programs, and this is just the overview of nursing. Keep in mind that the amount of knowledge that is required in nursing is massive.

It takes some people longer to master techniques than others, but with persistence and the proper attitude, the processes will eventually become second nature. Be prepared to learn something new every day; the opportunities to do so aren't usually difficult to find. Remember, mastering the processes of nursing is a process in itself. Take it one step at a time, and one day at a time. Someday the processes involved in the practice of nursing will become as easy as getting dressed.

Nurses are held accountable for thousands of procedures, and it is impractical to think that any one person can master every single procedure that can or will be performed. The more practical experience gained, the easier mastering new procedures will become. The art and science behind mastering nursing procedures can be compared to a spider's web, where every strand in the web has a beginning and an end, and every ending has a purpose. In a spider's web, there are hundreds, even thousands, of interconnected segments. The strands in the web change directions, create new paths, and have an almost infinite number of combinations from which to choose. To continue the analogy, every strand affects other strands—constructing more strands strengthens the web, each one contributing to a stronger foundation.

Some procedures begin at the same point, but somewhere down the line, each one may require a change in direction, and lead to new results. Beginning steps get mastered first because of repetition. For instance, before starting an IV, a sterile field must be created. Creating a sterile field is a part of numerous procedures. After mastering the procedure for creating sterile fields, nurses can move on to other parts of the procedure. With this in mind, the nurse only has to learn the new procedures from that point forward. Most procedures contain elements that are already familiar. For instance, starting a PICC line contains almost all of the same elements as starting an IV, but inserting a PICC line has a few extra steps along with extra equipment. Up to a point they are both the same, and then the two processes diverge. Starting an IV is considered the base knowledge for learning how to start a PICC line. Starting a PICC line is considered an advanced skill, but it cannot be learned until starting an IV is mastered. It is this knowledge base that will eventually lead to mastering more advanced skills.

In a more formal context, the process described above is known as scaffolding, meaning to build on something that is already known in order to reach a conclusion that is not yet known. In essence, this is a huge part of being a nurse: taking the training acquired in nursing school, building on it with experience and practice, and applying that knowledge in the field of nursing. This is the most common path to becoming proficient in the job and mastering processes.

Caring

Alongside the processes and tasks that are required, providing patients with care is necessary. Patient care comes in many forms and can be viewed in three areas: physical, mental, and emotional. Caring is an important part of being a nurse. If patients are not cared for in both the physical and psychological senses, it will be viewed as doing a sub-par job. These criteria set the tone for patient encounters and outcomes.

Nurses in general are constantly being evaluated. Patients are not the only people who will judge a nurse. Doctors, other nurses, supervisors, and patients' families are all included in the pool of people that evaluate a nurse's performance by the level of care that he or she provides. Constant evaluation is part of the daily work life, and evaluations come in two different forms. The first type of evaluation is made by the nurse when evaluating the patient's needs and determining how to meet those needs. The second form of evaluation is made by others such as: coworkers, doctors, family members, and the patients. This type of evaluation is based on the nurse's decisions and the care that is being provided. Both forms of the aforementioned evaluations are based on the degree of care or level of caring being provided.

Caring by Definition

There are numerous philosophies, theories, concepts, and practices that focus on the best way to care for and provide patients with care. Some choose to define patient care practice as a science and treat it as such. This type of practical nursing can also be called General System Theory, often defined as taking apart something that is whole and breaking it down into its parts to understand how those parts work together in a system. This theory is based on science and leads to the concept of science-based care. This type of care often leaves out the nurturing factor of providing care.

Another type of practical theory is called Adaptation Theory. This theory presents the idea that humans adapt on three levels: the self or internal adaptation, social adaptation to environment and others that surround them, and physical adaptation by biochemical processes. Adaptation Theory is broadly defined as the ability of the patient to adapt physically to the environment and other living things through interaction and response. Even though a nurse may not formally subscribe to this theory, it does influence a nurse in some form during his or her career. Adaptation is one of the processes that new nurses must recognize. Make note of things to do and things not to do, and get to know the quirks of coworkers and patients. This will be extremely helpful in your interactions with them, and a good indication that you are engaged and concerned.

The last theory offered here is the Developmental Theory that outlines the predictable and orderly development and growth that starts at conception and ends at death. The development and growth of humans are defined by factors such as environment, experience, emotions, genetics and heredity, and health.

Each of the three nursing theories mentioned above have four common concepts:

- the patient;
- the environment;
- the health of the patient;
- the nursing goals, roles, and functions.

The aforementioned theories are by no means an exhaustive list, and they are intended to be just a few representations of theory and practice to help illustrate the following idea. No matter what theory a nurse subscribes to, in the end they all lead to the same goal of delivering patient care. Patient care best defines the job of being a nurse.

Conclusion

New nurses will gain insight into the field of nursing over time just like Richard did. Discussing the realities associated with the practice of nursing is not intended to be a deterrent or a scare tactic; instead, these observations are intended to be informational about what is expected after graduating school and beginning nursing full time. Even though Richard's first day was horrible from his point-of-view, he has maintained a long and successful career. In the pages that follow more advice, tips, and pointers will be given from seasoned healthcare professionals that will help new nurses as they begin a career.

-2-

Things Your Professor Should Have Told You

"Knowing is not enough; we must apply. Willing is not enough; we must do."
                              -Johann Wolfgang von Goethe

Introduction

This chapter is broken down into two sections. The first section covers some misconceptions and truths about nursing and offers some advice on how to deal with these situations through the use of the buddy system. The second section offers advice for nurses on how to take care of themselves while on the job. These advices stems from years of experience, and even though this chapter does not encompass all the knowledge the job requires, it does offer some tips that aren't commonly taught in nursing school.

SECTION I: THE TRUTH

Misconceptions

Most things taught in nursing schools are taught as best practices, and by the same token many of these best practices are not the same practices that are being used in hospitals, doctors' offices, or other places outside of the classroom. These best practices often end up being outside what is conventionally accepted as the norm when put into practice at various institutions. This is where the deficit between learning and practice lays. This deficit can either be viewed as good or bad; it really just depends on the perception of the person making the determination.

The point is that nursing school doesn't teach students everything they need to know about the job, and there will always be peculiarities in the workplace that may come as a surprise. To complicate matters even further, each workplace has its own way of accomplishing goals; in some cases each floor or unit will have its own specific way of completing tasks, even within the same hospital. Even further down the chain, each charge nurse will have personal preferences about how things should get done by the nurses under his or her supervision. At the end of this chain of differences, a new nurse is expected to sift through all of the various ways of practicing and formulate a personal way of doing the job that will coincide with the organization's policies and accepted practices. This is a hard task to accomplish due to the many variables involved with the learning curve. However, in time a new nurse will get the hang of how things work and will learn what is expected of them.

Due to the sheer magnitude of various nursing practices, hospital administrators, and protocols, there is no way a nursing education program can teach a nursing student everything the student will need to know. This is where the advice given in this book can be put to use in order to aid in a smoother transition from being a nursing student to being a nurse.

Reality

Each day in nursing will be an exciting adventure. New experiences will occur at an alarming rate. Things can and will change in an instant. Look for these changes, prepare for them, and be ready to face new challenges the moment they arrive. No nursing program can prepare a student for each and every challenge of the job.

Nursing schools tend to gravitate toward the glorious aspects of being a nurse, and they overlook the unpleasant aspects. Nursing students are often lead to believe that nurses can save the world one patient at a time. In reality, saving lives on a daily basis is hyperbolic in nature. This concept is often used as a motivational tool to get students into and through nursing school. Nurses can save lives, but so can doctors, surgeons, and pre-hospital care providers. In general, this is not the particular care need of the majority of a nurse's patients. The majority of nurses will not be put to the threshold of life or death situations daily. Emergencies do happen, and certain nursing jobs are exposed to more critical situations than others, but a nurse's daily routine will not generally require any immediate life-saving skills to be performed. The majority of the time spent nursing is administering medications, charting the care rendered for each patient, and doing other required paperwork. The remainder of the time is spent caring for physical and mental needs such as:

- food and drink;
- aiding with or performing hygiene for the patient;
- talking with the patients and/or the patients' families addressing psychological needs.

In reality, a nurse spends a lot more time emptying bedpans and Foley catheter bags than performing cardiopulmonary resuscitation. This is a fact. With this fact in mind, be prepared to do both even though disposing of bodily fluids is less glorious than giving a patient a second chance at life.

Restroom Breaks

There are many universal truths in nursing just as there are in any profession. One of these truths is the fact that restroom breaks are a rarity, and when taken it must be a well thought out and planned event. When a nurse enters the restroom and closes the door, who is in charge of the care of the patients? Who will answer the call button? Inevitably, the minute after entering the restroom is the minute when someone will need something; sometimes it gets so busy that there is not a moment to spare to take care of personal physical needs.

Eating

Just like restroom breaks, eating is another personal need that often gets lost during a normal workday. Nurses spend so much time caring for others that they often forget to take care of themselves. Rarely does one get to sit down and enjoy a full meal during a lunch break. Skipping meals should never be an option. Even if mealtime is an eat-now-and-taste-it-later situation, make the time to eat. Without energy, it is hard to be productive. This is where the buddy system can help. Make sure someone is available to cover patients while eating. Charge nurses are supposed to ensure that nurses get breaks and are supposed to give nurses ample time to eat. This is not always the case. Even when charge nurses are good at providing coverage for breaks and eating, it doesn't always end up the way a nurse would like. Sometimes it just isn't possible to take a full break.

The Buddy System

Establishing the buddy system is one good way to prepare for restroom breaks and eating. Even though patients are assigned to a single nurse for their care, teamwork should always be utilized in the workplace. Pitch in and help other nurses when possible. In turn, other nurses will come and help out when you need it, including the tasks that take more than one person to accomplish. Since coverage is needed when the time comes for a break to eat, use the restroom, or for other personal reasons, the person chosen in the buddy system should be reliable and dependable.

The entire process is easier when someone is found that is trustworthy and dependable and will take care of patients as expected. Achieving the ability to eat in peace without the nagging worry that patients are getting neglected is a goal worth pursuing. On the other hand, if unreliable backup is used bad situations can appear in a hurry. If a patient makes a request to the nurse that is providing coverage and that nurse doesn't fulfill that request, the assigned nurse gets the blame. The blame always falls back on the nurse that is originally in charge of that patient's care. This is one reason why choosing a reliable buddy is so important. Finding someone whose professionalism is closely aligned to one's own is the key to success in picking a buddy. Basically, be careful not to select a slacker to be a buddy or the slacker's bad habits will then become the nurse's problems as well.

SECTION II: TAKING CARE OF YOU

Food

Keep an extra supply of healthy snacks and quick backup foods on hand. Don't be tempted by the cookies in the break room. Yes, they may be filling, but after the sugar wears off, hunger and lack of energy set in again. This is counterproductive. Plan to have quick snacks available for instances where time is crucial and in short supply. When it is not possible to break away from patient care, a quick snack can really help keep energy levels up. The snack can be carried in a pocket, a handbag, back pack, or stored in a locker if available. Where the snack is kept is not as important as the fact that one is available. There are several items that nurses should have quick access to, food is one and clothes are another.

Uniforms

It is a good idea to have a complete change of clothes on hand and readily available for times of need, and there are many reasons behind this advice. One reason is if a uniform gets soiled during the course of a normal workday, having a backup on hand will prove to be useful because the nurse can quickly change uniforms and carry on. If a clean uniform is not available, patients will cringe at the sight of a nurse walking around with blood-covered scrubs. It is unsanitary, and it runs the risk of spreading disease and germs from one patient to another. In some instances, if a backup uniform is not available when a uniform becomes soiled, the nurse will be sent home. This type of situation should be avoided as it causes undue stress among the entire workforce. Loss of pay is one issue for the unprepared, and increasing the workload on coworkers is another. Also, the charge nurse will not be pleased because of the loss of the nurse if the nurse is sent home.

Another good reason for having a backup uniform available is the risk of being required to stay beyond the normal work schedule due to unforeseen "states of emergency" such as inclement weather or a mass casualty incident. If any of these occurrences happen, an extra uniform to change into will be nice. These occurrences don't happen on a regular basis, but that fact shouldn't be an excuse to be unprepared for the situation when it arises. To give a context for this advice, the following story illustrates why an extra uniform is important.

Cathy's Lesson

It was my second week on the job. I was new and I was still in awe and shock of the fact that I was a nurse and how much I didn't know. That morning, I had just completed my initial rounds on five patients when Nancy, the senior nurse on the floor, stepped out of one her patient's room and asked for some help. Nancy needed me to help her clean up one of her patients. I can say that this was not appealing to me at the time, but being the new kid on the block, it was my time to earn some brownie points. I knew that the right thing to do was to agree without hesitation, and that's just what I did.

She told me, "It will only take a minute," and asked me to grab some linens. She added, "Don't go in without me. Just wait for me here." That should have been my first clue, but at the time I didn't think anything about it. So, I went and got some clean linens and returned to the room and stood patiently just outside the door. As I stood there a strange odor surrounded me. I shuffled over to the other side of the hall, but it didn't help. The odor was over there too. I tried holding my breath, but it was no use. Each time I breathed, I would catch a whiff of the most horrific smell that I had ever encountered in my life. I could only think of one thing, "What died?"

Nancy came back down the hall holding two yellow masks and some hospital issue toothpaste. I must have looked like a confused and 'trying not to gag' idiot, and I'm sure the dumb look on my face conveyed my thoughts.

Nancy handed me a mask and instructed me to place the toothpaste on the inside of the mask. She quickly recognized another one of my dumb looks. She explained, "It will help with the smell. You will smell the toothpaste instead of the feces we are about to clean up." Then it clicked in my head. I did as I was told and was willing to try anything. The smell was really getting to me. I wasn't looking forward to going into that patient's room. I reasoned to myself, "if it is this bad out here, I can't imagine what it's going to be like inside the room."

We went in. My eyes started watering a little bit. I could smell toothpaste and feces, but it was bearable. I didn't even want to think about how bad the smell would have been without my toothpaste barrier. Nancy insisted on being the one that would turn the 300-pound man. This didn't make any sense to me as she was only five feet tall and maybe a hundred pounds soaking wet, but she was in charge of this patient. Given the responsibility of being the "cleaner," I watched as Nancy used leverage and proper body mechanics to turn the patient over on his side.

This is when I went to work. I was gloved and masked trying only to breathe through my mouth. I rolled the sheets just as she instructed me. I was trying to contain the liquid stench. As I made my first attempt, Nancy blurted out, "careful around the firing hole." As luck would have it, it was too late; the "firing pin" had been activated. The semi-formed feces shot out faster than a speeding bullet. With force and speed, the brown liquid flew across the bed soaking my scrub bottoms, running down my legs soaking my socks and shoes, and finally splashing on the floor. In disgust, I finished cleaning the patient and retreated into the nurse's locker room in an effort to decontaminate myself.

I learned several valuable lessons that day. First, when given the opportunity to be the person turning the patient instead of the one cleaning the patient, my advice is to take it. Second, always keep a complete change of clothes on hand at work or in the car.

Concluding Cathy's Lesson

Cathy's advice is solid and should be taken to heart. There is no way to know when an accident will happen, and being prepared for such an incident is prudent. Note that Cathy advises to keep a "complete change of clothes" on hand. A complete change of clothes is defined as tops, bottoms, socks, under garments, and shoes. This is good advice and shouldn't be underestimated.

Shoes

Shoes are important. Shoes are a nurse's best friend. Being on the go for the majority of a twelve-hour shift can seem like an eternity with aching feet. Since every person is different, it would be futile to try and tell any given person the best way to take care of his or her own feet. So, little advice can be offered about the type of shoe that works best. This is a personal choice that must ultimately be decided on by the wearer. Just make sure that the shoes can and will offer comfort and support for twelve hours, and then get three pairs.

Alternate wearing two pairs of shoes during the course of the week and keep the third pair available as part of the backup uniform. By alternating shoes every other day, feet will remain in a state of flux, and it also increases the longevity of the shoes by not putting constant stress on the same places of the insoles. After a while, the shoes will mold to one's feet. At this point, it is time to begin looking for a new pair, or at least get ready to replace the insoles. This can happen as quickly as six months depending on wear. It never hurts to check with an expert when determining if the shoes are worn out. Many shoe retailers offer this service free of charge. Simply take the shoes into the retailer and have them inspected.

Shoes molding to one's feet is very different than being broken in. A broken-in shoe provides comfort and gives the wearer support where needed and bends in all the right places according to the wearer's feet. Molding means that when looking down inside of the shoe, the outline of the foot imprinted on the insole can be seen. If the shoes are still in good shape, simply buy a new pair of comfortable insoles. Foot care is essential.

Personal Care

Along with making sure that a complete uniform is available, having personal hygiene products available—in the event that extended work becomes necessary—should be a part of personal care preparedness not to be overlooked. This means having an emergency kit of some sort. In the kit, the nurse will want to make sure to have the following items available:

- hair care products, such as combs, brushes, and shampoo;
- oral care products, such as dental floss, toothpaste, a tooth brush, and mouthwash;
- deodorant;
- any medication necessary for at least a 48-hour period, which includes prescription medications, over the counter medications, and headache pills; and
- female nurses should make sure they have feminine hygiene products.

Taking hospital medications is usually against policy, and this practice isn't recommended as this can lead to trouble, such as getting terminated. Furthermore, taking any of the aforementioned items is frowned upon as this is considered stealing.

Being prepared will make it that much easier to maintain a positive attitude, and it offers the ability to deal with any unforeseen situations when they occur. Even though regular shifts can be 8-12 hours, there may be times when working longer shifts is required.

Conclusion

The ideas presented in this chapter are a few pointers that can make the workday just a little better. This is not an inclusive list, nor is it intended to be, but this advice is based on the experience of seasoned nurses. As stated before, there is no way to completely prepare a first-year nurse for the demands of the job, but the ideas above will help. Ultimately, this knowledge is left in the hands of the individual. Each person must decide what knowledge is useful and what knowledge isn't. Through the experience and advice of others, a better perspective on how to prepare for the job can be achieved.

-3-

Listening

"The most important practical lesson that can be given to nurses is to teach them what to observe."

-Florence Nightingale

Introduction

Peers, doctors, patients, and patients' families are constantly judging nurses. The terms "good nurse" and "bad nurse" are used to label the overall abilities of the nurse. One factor that contributes to this "labeling" is the ability to listen. In general, the judgment is made through the perception of a nurse's ability to listen, understand, and interpret what exactly is being said. Listening skills are often talked about and sometimes even emphasized, but the skills involved in listening are hardly ever explained. The following information will give added insight into listening.

Communication Cycle

The ability to listen stretches far beyond the ability to hear audible noise; it leans more toward a concept than a physical ability. Listening is actually the part of the communication cycle known as decoding. The communication cycle basics are as follows:

1. The sender—also known as the speaker—encodes the message, which means he or she prepares the communication through thinking about it.

2. Then the sender verbalizes the message to the receiver—who is also known as the person to whom the sender is speaking.

3.   The receiver then decodes the message, which means they hear the message and formulate an interpretation of the message.

The ability to formulate the meaning of messages plays an important role in nursing. It is easy to misinterpret messages due to the vastness of information that is conveyed on a daily basis. Inevitably, any misinterpretation trickles down to the patients, and this usually ends in adverse consequences both for the nurse and the patient.

In an effort to avoid miscommunication, mastering listening skills should be a priority. Understanding that communication is extremely important and should always be at the forefront of any interaction in the workplace will be a tremendous aid in job performance. In order to perform assigned duties appropriately, the nurse must fully understand what is expected (and asked) of him or her by other nurses, doctors, and patients. For instance, if a doctor scribbles an order that is not legible in a patient's chart, never make an educated guess as to what the order says. Always get clarification on any order that is unclear before moving on with any procedure or the administration of any medication.

Active Listening

Learning to be an "active listener" is a process, and listed next are eight key elements that can aid nurses in the process of becoming better active listeners. Being an active listener requires a person to:

1.   Stop talking and do not make any premature responses. Talking while listening is virtually impossible.

2.   Have patience. Allow the speaker to complete his or her thoughts without interruptions. Wait for the speaker to finish speaking; never talk over the person, and never finish someone else's thoughts.

3.   Prepare to listen to a speaker by focusing all attention on the speaker, and try to avoid distractions. It is easy to get sidetracked during a conversation, but stay focused on the message.

4.   Always keep in mind that body language plays a key role in communication. When listening, don't shuffle papers, look at a watch, or act anxious by moving around unnecessarily. These kinds of gestures suggest to the speaker that the listener's mind is somewhere else instead of focusing on the conversation.

5.   As a listener, learn to interpret cues from the speaker's body language, and try to pick up on what is left unsaid. Listening also involves one's eyes and not just ears. Often times, what isn't being said is just as important—if not more—than what is being said.

6.   Being a good listener involves the ability to understand the big picture and the intended

meaning of the message rather than just hearing the words that are being delivered by the speaker.

7. Tone and volume can be an indicator from the speaker on how the message should be received.

8. Never be judgmental about the speaker's ability to communicate. Sometimes it takes some people longer to get their words right before speaking, and be patient when listening to people speak in order to gain a better understanding of the message.

This list is not intended to fully educate a nurse on how to become a good listener, but it is a good starting point to build on through research, practice, and experience.

The following story is a real experience that a female patient had in an emergency room, and it is intended to demonstrate how being a good listener can prevent adverse effects on a patient.

DEBBY'S SAGA
Debby's Situation

The background information on the patient is as follows: the female patient has Short Bowel Syndrome, and she is currently under the care of a surgeon and a nutritional doctor. The patient underwent a surgical step-procedure to lengthen her bowel, which was a success and lengthened her bowel to approximately 100cm in length. As a result of her condition, the patient has a high-output ileostomy even after her bowel had been lengthened. Her output ranges vastly depending on her intake of fluids and food. At any point during the patient's treatment it is not uncommon for her ileostomy to output 11 liters of fluid in a single 24-hour period.

At the time of one such incident, the patient was on total parenteral nutrition (TPN) of 2000 ml infused over 12 hours with a one-hour ramp up and a one-hour ramp down time. Also, she is allowed to intake as much fluid and food orally as she wants. Being on TPN is the answer to getting the patient the much needed nutrition in a form that her body can absorb since she cannot properly absorb nutrition through her digestive tract. The patient has been on TPN for approximately two years, and the TPN is delivered through a Hickman port that was placed by her surgeon. Both the TPN and the maintenance of the Hickman port are managed by a home health service that visits the patient weekly.

Due to the shortness of her bowel and the associated absorption problems that coincide with her illness, the patient has a high hemodynamic sensitivity. She is dependent on her oral fluid intake and the TPN, as she is prone to severe dehydration and electrolyte imbalances within a matter of hours if her routine gets interrupted. If the patient goes twenty-four hours without TPN, she has been known to reach critical levels in her potassium and magnesium count. Also, the telltale signs of her dehydration are severe muscle cramps, nausea, and sometimes violent vomiting. It only takes a matter of hours for this to occur, as she is an atypical case due to her complicated history. Due to the fact that her condition is outside the general parameters of standard medicine, it is hard for healthcare workers to understand her condition and accept the facts that go along with it.

Debby's Incident

As the story begins, one night at approximately 8:30 pm, 30 minutes after starting her TPN, the patient's Hickman port ruptured. Her husband, having been through this event previously, clamped the line with the in-line clamp. Then, he wrapped and taped the ruptured portion with sterile gauze. He then called the on-call physician from his wife's doctor's office that advised them to go to the emergency room. The doctor stated that she must be seen and evaluated by a physician. They got in the car and drove to the hospital as directed by the doctor, and they arrived at approximately 10:30 pm. The patient lives an hour away from the hospital. Due to the specialized nature of her illness, this is the closest hospital that can care for her condition. Without traveling out of the state, the patient has no other alternative hospital.

The patient was triaged in the emergency room, and around 1:30 am she was finally brought into a room. The doctor came in and evaluated the patient by obtaining her history and current situation. The doctor left and said she was going to put in orders. Shortly after 2:30 am, the nurse made her first appearance in the patient's room. By this time, the patient was having severe cramps, and she had received no treatment whatsoever. The couple tried to explain the situation to the nurse. They told the nurse that the patient was dehydrated and needed fluids in a hurry. The nurse interrupted and said, "there is no way she is dehydrating that fast." Needless to say, the non-caring callousness of this assessment by this unknowing nurse did not sit well with either the patient or her husband. The nurse left the room saying she would "go and get things." A different nurse came in about 10 minutes later to start an IV. The doctor came in later and asked why the husband wanted to see her, asking, "is it because nothing has been done yet?" The reply was obviously yes and included the fact that the first nurse that came into the room essentially called the couple liars and then left. The two then requested that the original nurse not be allowed back in the room. The doctor responded by saying that she would have the charge nurse come by and speak with them, which never happened.

Around 3:00 am, the patient finally received fluids, pain medications for her cramping, and her initial labs drawn. By this point, the patient had been without any IV fluids for nineteen hours, and was at a 1,100 ml deficit from her TPN. Dehydration was occurring and confirmed by the doctor via lab results. After the fluids were started, the patient's cramps eventually subsided with time and treatment. Upon the doctor's reassessment, the doctor stated that the patient's lab work was abnormal and that there would be treatments to correct the situation.

Debby's Outcome

Three days later, the Hickman port was placed and the patient was discharged from the hospital. Two weeks later, the patient's lab readings were back into the range that they had been prior to the incident.

It has been the patient's experience that the average nurse is unprepared to treat her unique condition, as it does not fall into a usual category. In this case, the time delay and fluid disruption created an imbalance that took weeks to return back to normal levels. This situation could have been avoided if the nurse would have listened to the patient and given her the fluids she needed in a timely fashion.

Unfortunately, this was not an isolated incident. Debby had similar experiences on at least two other occasions at the same hospital.

Conclusion

Debby is not alone in her experience, as others have suffered as a result from nurses and doctors refusing to listen or just outright ignoring them. Patients and family members have been dismissed as uneducated and overreacting to medical conditions. People that are chronically sick battle the illnesses for years. These people have extensive experience with the problems associated with the condition because the problem is dealt with on a daily basis. The patients and family members know what works for the patient and what doesn't. They become experts on the illness. These people realize they are special cases, but it is frustrating when the doctors and nurses summarily dismiss personal experience and knowledge.

These kinds of incidents can be avoided when proper listening skills are practiced. It seems like this should be common sense and, in a way, it is. Listening should come naturally, but this isn't always the case. Being a good listener requires effort, training, and experience.

Choosing not to be an active listener will result in poor patient outcomes and will damage the trust relationship between patient and nurse. Listening should be a part of every patient care plan. Listening skills are not mandated nor can they be enforced, but if patient care is the focus, the nurse will listen to what the patient is saying and respond accordingly.

-4-

Workflow

"Bound by paperwork, short on hands, sleep, and energy... nurses are rarely short on caring."
-Sharon Hudacek

Introduction

The industry standard for patient-to-nurse ratio is supposed to be 6:1. Some days that may be the case, but some days it isn't. Some days the assignment load reaches ten patients. Those days aren't going to be easy ones. Nevertheless, figuring out how to best meet the needs of each patient is part of the job. A great mnemonic that aids in dealing with planning are the five Ps: Prior Planning Prevents Poor Performance. Having a plan for the day can help prevent a disaster. Even if the plan is destined to fail—and sometimes the plan will fail—this should not be an excuse for not being prepared to deal with the day and the patient workload. Without a plan, patient care will suffer, stress levels will increase, and a nurse will have a horrible day, only to be topped by the next shift when the nurse gets assigned eleven patients.

The Plan

One way to prevent chaos and avoid patient neglect is by organizing the patient load into a workflow. A workflow is the mode in which patient care is delivered in the least amount of trips. Devising a workflow is important for many reasons. One reason is that time spent standing and walking leads to a lack of energy, and a lack of energy poses the risk of making mistakes. Patient safety should always be at the forefront of each nurse and patient encounter and creating a workflow helps in addressing this issue.

Setting up a workflow should always include the element of patient safety, and this is just one factor to consider. Other things that should be considered in planning a workflow are:

- diagnosis and co-morbidities;
- physical abilities and disabilities;
- family support;
- specialized needs or testing.

Additionally, in creating a workflow, plan for times of routine labs and serial x-rays, noting whether the test will be done at the bedside or if there is a need for the patient to go to a specific department to have the test completed.

The items listed above are just a few ideas that need addressing in developing a workload routine. Experience and daily demands will eventually become the deciding factors when developing a workflow that works best for each nurse and shift; the advice above offers a good starting place.

Starting the Day

When a nurse makes initial rounds, that round will dictate the workflow for the majority of the shift with the exception of discharges and new admissions. The idea to remember concerning workflow is to always be flexible. No one can ever account for everything that might arise during a shift—the best laid plans can quickly go awry. Murphy's Law dictates that anything that can go wrong will go wrong—the same applies to nursing. Changes are a major part of the daily work in the field of nursing. Changes occur in an instant and must be dealt with in a timely and efficient manner. Expect the change, and don't be shocked when it happens. Instead, focus on the task at hand. This benefits both the nurse and the patient by working through problems without outside interruptions. Problems often arise that a nurse cannot control, and a "go with the flow" attitude goes a long way.

Preventing diminishing health of a patient is a primary concern, and steps can be taken to prevent diminishing health. The following ideas will help in this matter. At the beginning of each shift there will be a period of time when the previous nurse gives a hand-off/shift change report. This is the opportunity for a nurse to start the organization process. Gathering information is part of the prevention process, and it helps with creating a workflow. When the on-coming nurse gets the patient reports from the previous nurse, there are key elements to note and certain questions to ask:

- Which patients have drains, if any?
- Which patients are restrained?
- Which patients are on pain management?

- Which patients have specific nutritional needs (especially for those patients that have diabetes)?
- Are any of the patients pre- or post-op?
- Are there any patients with isolation requirements?
- Are there any patients with an altered mental status?
- Are there any patients with other special needs?
- What is the ambulatory status that coincides with a fall-risk assessment?

Also, don't forget to ask about the patients' support networks. Inquiring about family members, friends, or any special religious needs that should be addressed will be beneficial in the patients' care plans. Understanding patients' support systems will ultimately provide a better overall understanding of patients' needs, and aid in determining the workflow for the shift. By having a well-prepared plan, a nurse gains the ability to deal with situations when they arise and often prevents them from ever occurring.

Rounds

After gathering information from the hand-off/shift change report, it is time to start the initial round. There are many different ways to start initial rounds. One common error often made is getting bogged down with the tasks at the beginning of the shift. Tasks shouldn't be performed during the initial round unless it is deemed an emergency. The initial round should be quick. It should be performed in the manner of a triage system. This allows for getting an idea of the immediate needs of the patients. Next, choosing a starting point based on the report helps begin the development of a workflow process for the day. Start by going to the most acute patient first.

After entering the sickest patient's room, perform a rapid observation determining the patient's stability or instability. When done with this observation, and after correcting any immediate issues, move on to the next patient in order of severity. Continue on in this process and keep in mind that the last patient to assess is the patient that needs more emotional support than patients requiring labor-intensive care. Getting caught in a room by an elderly patient that wants to share his or her life story can severely hinder the process of caring for other patients that have more immediate needs, such as pain management or other medication administration. After attending to all the patients' physical needs, return to fulfill the emotional needs of these patients. Sometimes getting caught in a patient's room cannot be avoided, and when this happens, make a polite excuse and move on to the next situation while remembering not to make promises that cannot or will not be kept.

Prevention

After establishing the safety portion of the patients' needs during the initial round, move on to preventive measures:

- check the patency and stability of IVs and drains;
- confirm that fall prevention measures are in place where needed;
- check to assure that restraints are in place, working correctly, and not too tight.

While performing these tasks, make a mental list to delegate tasks to support staff as needed. As part of the team, the support staff needs to be aware of situations to look out for while delivering patient care.

Medication Administration

After confirming that all the patients are safe and are not experiencing anything adverse, move on to medications. Medication organization should come only after completing initial rounds because there is always the possibility that a patient will have a pressing issue that needs immediate attention, such as finding a patient in respiratory distress. The initial round will reveal anything that needs immediate attention.

When beginning medication administration, start with either the PRN—as needed—medications and give them out as needed or requested, or start with the patients who only need PO—by mouth—medications. This helps with the workflow by avoiding getting tied up in the administration of more complicated medications.

Devise a way of giving medications that will maintain an order. Start with the patient who needs the most medications or with the patient who needs the fewest medications. Either way, give medications to only one patient at a time. This will prevent errors. Don't try to give all the PO medications in one round, and then come back to give intravenous medications in a separate round. This is a bad idea. This practice is confusing, and the opportunity for error increases. One practical way is to start with the patient that only needs PO medications. By doing this, the risk of infiltrating an IV is avoided (also known as blowing a vein). An infiltration falls into the task-oriented care mentioned earlier, and these situations will only slow down the workflow.

By ending the medication rounds with the complicated patient, the workflow will maintain consistency. A patient that has multiple medications given through multiple routes is labor intensive. By saving the complicated patient until last, time is saved and falling behind in medication administration is circumvented. Also, take an extra minute with those complicated patients to look for contraindications and side effects of the medications, and be familiar with antidotes. Always keep a supply of flushes, alcohol wipes, gloves, tape, and scissors readily available, as this practice will pay dividends in time conservation and efficiency.

Giving medications requires preparedness. Just as with anything in nursing, medication administration requires a plan; poor planning equals poor results. One way to prepare is to always make sure to have water available for PO medications. Walking into a patient's room with a handful of pills and no water is bad. Besides wasting time by having to go back out of the room to get water, the patient may deem the nurse incompetent and not focused as a result. During the PO medication round, prepare a water cart and leave the cart just outside the room for quick access when necessary. Also, have some snacks on the cart, as some medications should be taken with food. Even if a cart is not prepared, always make sure food and water is available when administering pills and other PO medications.

When administering medications, the five "rights" need to be checked. This mnemonic is used as a safety measure, and its usage should never be taken lightly. In order to assure accuracy, make sure to have the:

1.   Right patient.
2.   Right drug.
3.   Right dose.
4.   Right route.
5.   Right amount.

This is paramount in assuring that a mistake doesn't occur. Also, confirm the availability of the medications. It doesn't happen often, but there are instances when the hospital runs out of certain medications due to unforeseen events, such as a national shortage, a recall on medications, or the ordering doctor is unfamiliar with the formulary in the pharmacy.

Take a Break

Once the medication rounds are completed, it is a good time for a break. Go to the bathroom, and get something to drink. The patients have been cared for, and now it is the nurse's turn. Breaks should be part of the workflow plan and should be taken advantage of when possible. Oftentimes, breaks get neglected because nurses get too busy caring for patients. Without recharging a battery, it will stop working; take a minute and recharge your batteries.

Charting

After the break, follow up on any additional charting requirements. Some systems are "scan and give." This system automatically charts any medication given once it is scanned, but even the best system does not make notes for the nurse. So, make sure to keep up with charting requirements as soon as possible. Remember that at any given moment, things can fall apart, and trying to remember details hours later will be difficult if not impossible. Even the most brilliant minds will forget something.

Tasks

Before getting tied up in complex task-oriented care, make one more quick round to patients' rooms, give some comfort care, and tie up any loose ends, or work will begin to pile up. After this, get ready to begin the task-oriented procedures. Stock up on supplies; gather any and all equipment needed including—but not limited to—replacement or back up supplies. This prevents having to run all the way back to the supply room if something is dropped. Do all of this before entering the patient's room. Nothing annoys a patient worse than an unprepared nurse. Try to make each visit a one-time deal, and then move on to the next patient. This relieves the pressure of having to return to complete an unfinished task. If a patient needs extra attention, try to get some coverage for the other patients and coordinate efforts with the backup so that the both of you are not tied up with labor-intensive tasks at the same time. Dressing changes cannot be abandoned, so backup is not always available. Plan for help when needed, and have a backup plan for that plan. Planning cannot be stressed enough as it is the backbone of performance. Make a plan, implement the plan, and be flexible enough to change when the plan isn't working.

Teamwork

Teamwork is key when trying to plan out the day and assuring that all the needed tasks can be accomplished in the shift. Remember that a nurse is part of a team, and nurses don't have to do everything alone. This is the reason why hospitals hire support personnel. Support personnel such as techs are there to help when needed, and nurses shouldn't hesitate to use them. Also, in this instance, the buddy system should be based on geography and the acuity of the patients. This will help when aid is needed in a hurry. Don't just pick anybody to help out. Make sure that person is capable of providing the correct help when needed. If the helper doesn't have the ability, knowledge, or skills to help then that person isn't really any help at all in critical situations.

The following story illustrates the process that Manny went through in order to find a workflow that worked best for him.

Manny's Lesson

Veteran nurse Manny recounts how he struggled to find a workflow that worked best for him and how he learned from his colleagues.

I worked the night shift on the second floor at my brand new job in the hospital. At the time, I had only been out of school for two months and on the job for two weeks. I struggled a bit at first as I tried to fit in with my coworkers. They weren't very helpful either. I had my suspicions that Lucy, my preceptor at the hospital, had already poisoned any chance of them liking me. Lucy was a crotchety old nag that wasn't one for polite conversation. She would snap my head off in an instant every time she saw me do something that wasn't to her liking. She was more of a trial-and-error sort of teacher rather than helpful. I began wondering why she was even a nurse. If nurses are supposed to be caring and kind, I couldn't see any evidence of it in her at all. I was sure that she was talking bad about me behind my back. By the end of my first week on the job, I had already become defensive, and I started making my own judgments about my coworkers.

That first week was hard, and I remember thinking to myself, "I seem to be the only nurse doing any work in this place." Every time I walked by the nurses' station, they were all sitting there laughing and talking. The charge nurse seemed to be the ringleader. The other nurses were there along with the respiratory therapist; it looked like a party, and I wasn't invited to join in on the conversation. One night I had passed the desk four times and every time it was the same; they were all sitting around enjoying themselves. On my fifth pass, I overheard one of my colleagues say, "Should we tell 'em?" Then, I heard the charge nurse respond, "Not yet, let's see if it's a new record." Then, there was a bit of chuckling.

Needless to say, this pissed me off to no end. I fumed as I continued my numerous treks to and from the medication room, supply room, clean utility room, nutrition refrigerator, and my personal favorite, the soiled utility room. As I worked my tail off, I again thought to myself, "Why are those nurses so lazy? All they do is sit at that desk all night making fun of me."

On my sixth journey by the desk, I heard some laughter, some snickering, and one of them say, " I can't take it anymore, let's help him out." Someone agreed and they called me over. The charge nurse piped up and informed me that I have set a new floor record for a graduate nurse. Puzzled and pissed, I stated, "I don't understand."

One of the nurses reached under the desk, and she pulled out a gift bag with a big blue bow tied around the handles of the bag. She stretched her arm out toward me and said, "Here. This is your award." I hesitated for a minute as I realized that everyone was staring at me. Eventually, I took the bag from her. "Open it," she said.

I untied the bow, and then I reached down into the bag and pulled out a pair of baby shoes. The look on my face must have been quite a sight. I can only imagine my look of confusion mixed with embarrassment. To make matters worse, everyone burst out laughing. When the laughter settled, I looked at the charge nurse and said, "What are these for?"

She answered, "The award is for the most grossly inefficient way to handle your workload. You've probably walked ten miles tonight going back and forth needlessly. Those shoes are a symbol. The baby needs to learn to walk." I knew this must have some underlying meaning that I did not yet understand. Over the next twenty minutes, I learned more about being a nurse than I did during my entire nursing school program. I have never forgotten those lessons from that day.

It turned out that Lucy, my angry preceptor, had been talking with the other nurses. As a result, they had devised a way of helping me to understand the intricacies of being a nurse. They each took turns at giving me a piece of advice. Each one was different, yet they all were useful.

I still remember the lessons, and I practice them on a daily basis. By sharing my knowledge, I hope that new nurses will find some useful ideas they can use as well. The advice listed below is in no particular order, and is simple and practical:

- If a patient is incontinent, put a bunch of linens in the room at once. This way you don't have to make a special trip to the linen closet each time the soiled sheets need changing.

- Get a penlight. This way you don't wake a patient up every time you do rounds or check an IV. A sleeping patient is a happy patient.

- Don't wear squeaky shoes. This also wakes patients up.

- Fill all the water pitchers at once. This way water is always available when giving meds or when the patient wants a drink.

- If you have to take a rectal temperature, warm the lubrication up first. The patient will thank you in the end. (Pun intended).

- Always wear scrubs that have pockets. In your pockets keep extra alcohol/chloraprep wipes, IV flushes, sterile 2x2s, and tape. This keeps unnecessary trips to the supply room to a minimum. Remember to restock these items often.

- Keep a set of gloves in your pocket at all times. One never knows when an IV will decide to fall out or some other bodily fluid incident might occur. If the glove box happens to be empty, you are in trouble.
- Don't be afraid to ask for help. Teamwork is a must, and that is what technicians are for. Don't abuse them, but use them when needed.
- Don't make unnecessary trips. Do as much as you can in one trip.
- Plan ahead, and remember that prevention is always a time saver in the long run.

I now know that the nurses weren't intentionally trying to be mean to me. They were actually trying to let me figure things out for myself, and when they saw that I just wasn't getting it; they stepped in and offered me sound advice. At the time, I hated them for the callousness, but after I found out that there was a method to the madness, I was a better nurse because of it. I guess this was some sort of right-of-passage training. They let me learn the hard way. At the time, I wasn't very happy with the ordeal, but I soon learned how valuable the advice they gave me was in helping me find a rhythm. I also learned not to be so quick to judge things based on appearance. The nurses weren't being lazy. Instead, they had learned how to manage their workflows. To the untrained eye—

which was mine at the time—it only appeared they were being lazy and not working. Fifteen years later, a new nurse might say the same thing about me because I have learned how to find a flow, which gives me some time to rest on occasions by saving me countless hours of unnecessary activity. My job is so much easier now than it was in the beginning because the other nurses helped me to find my own workflow.

Conclusion

New nurses can apply the lessons that Manny learned as they begin to figure out their own workflow and what works best for them. Creating a workflow is important, and this process will take some time and effort. By understanding the basics of how to organize and manage a workflow, new nurses will have an easier transition from being a student to being a professional.

-5-

Mistakes

"We may encounter many defeats but we must not be defeated."

-Maya Angelou

Introduction

Mistakes happen. Mistakes are a natural part of being human. No matter how hard one tries, eventually a mistake will occur. Many of the mistakes made in life have few or little consequences. Unfortunately, when a nurse makes a mistake patients suffer and that is always a big deal. No matter the ranking in the grand scheme of life, big or small, mistakes made by nurses have an impact on patient outcomes. There is only one way to assure that a mistake doesn't affect a patient's outcome, and that is the act of prevention. To prevent the mistake from ever occurring is a goal that should always be at the forefront of a nurse's mind, but the act of prevention is much easier said than done. Prevention entails many facets that are time consuming and rely on careful consideration on a constant basis. In an already time-consuming and sometimes overwhelming job such as nursing, prevention can often times be overlooked. Ignoring prevention measures should never happen, but it does.

What are the most common types of mistakes? What are the outcomes after the mistake has been made? What can a nurse do to stop a mistake before the mistake ever happens? This chapter covers these topics and more in order to give nurses a better understanding of mistakes in relation to the job of nursing.

This chapter is broken down into three sections. The first section covers six common types of mistakes:

- Complete omissions
- Partial omissions
- Arrogance
- Intuition
- Assumption
- Communication

The second section lists the four classifications of mistakes:

- near misses,
- those that reach the patient without harm,
- those that reach the patient with harm, and
- catastrophic.

The third section's focus is on: prevention measures, the consequences after a mistake is made, and the emotional impact of mistakes on nurses.

SECTION I: TYPES OF MISTAKES

Mistakes that are made by nurses are classified into six general categories. The ability to recognize and identify these six types of mistakes will help nurses by making nurses aware of situations to avoid. Therefore, the first step in prevention is education.

Complete Omissions

A complete omission is when information is not passed on to the individuals charged with patient care. Complete omissions, either intentional or unintentional, can impact and/or hinder patient care. This type of mistake can be as simple as forgetting to tell a colleague, a family member, or oncoming staff about a patient's condition, previous medical history, or plan of care. In many instances, the family may not give you the whole story, the patient may withhold key information, or outgoing staff may forget to relay information. These types of mistakes all fall under the heading of a complete omission.

One scenario of a complete omission is when an elderly patient forgets to tell the nurse about the "water pill" that the patient takes every day in the morning. This omission may be either intentional or not. Either way, without this knowledge the nurses and doctors involved in that patient's care will not know to include the medication in the patient's plan of care. The patient's missed doses can lead to several different possible outcomes, none of which will be good. In the above example, the patient's lack of the diuretic can exacerbate her congestive heart failure and lead to respiratory distress or even future readmission post-discharge because this was just the trigger to a chronic situation.

Another, yet more complex example of a complete omission, is a patient that is unable to tell the nurse anything due to his or her medical condition such as a multi-system trauma patient that is unconscious. This example is not intentional on the patient's part, or anyone else's part for that matter, but it does happen and the outcomes from not knowing pertinent information can have severe consequences on patient outcomes. In the case of the complex trauma patient, information about his Coumadin therapy for a mitral valve replacement may not be detected for hours. This makes the needed surgery for the trauma patient high risk due to bleeding. In a true emergency, not knowing this valuable information can lead to death.

Again, complete omissions can have serious consequences such as disrupting the patient's treatment plan due to the missed medications, side effects, and contraindications. One way to prevent complete omissions requires a certain level of detective work. On a conscious patient this requires a thorough interview by asking the right questions that will prompt patients not to forget to disclose medication information such as, "Do you take any medications on a daily basis?" Learning to use follow up questions will also help, such as, "What medication do you take in the morning? Do you have a list? Are you due for any refills?" This is not intended to be a complete list, rather this is intended to make nurses aware that thorough interviewing can aid in warding off complete omissions. On an unconscious patient, prevention measures are not applicable.

Partial Omissions

A partial omission is similar to a complete omission, but it has slight variations. A partial omission is the incomplete sharing of information that affects patient outcomes or plan of care. Only getting half of the information can have the same consequences as not getting any information at all.

One example of partial omission is incomplete documentation of a performed procedure such as a dressing change on an IV site. After the procedure, the dressing is labeled with the date and time performed, but the nurse forgets to chart the procedure as completed in the medical record. The next nurse checks the chart and assumes that the dressing change has yet to be completed because it isn't in the chart. So, the nurse gather's all the supplies necessary to do the dressing change only to find out upon arrival at the patient's side that the procedure has already been completed. Even though this small event doesn't affect the patient's outcome, this situation has wasted valuable time and resources that could be better utilized elsewhere.

Partial omissions aren't necessarily generated from healthcare providers. Other influences are a factor in partial omissions. Family members can generate partial omissions as well. One such instance would be when a family member provides the name of the medication but not the dose. Not knowing the correct dose is a partial omission.

Another example, using the elderly patient's "water pill" stated earlier, the family member might tell the nurse that the elderly patient takes a little yellow pill twice a day, but doesn't know the dose. In this instance, the nurse doesn't know what the medication is or the dose of that mysterious yellow pill. Someone has to bring those pills in for evaluation or the prescribing physician has to be contacted. When this happens the nurse will have to play the part of a detective and track down the needed information. What can be learned from this? It is always a good idea to have a list of medications that state: names, dosage, and times administered. An instance such as this is a teaching moment, and this lesson can be relayed to the patient and his or her family. This is a prevention measure that not only saves time, but it wards off potential adverse effects.

Arrogance

Nothing is scarier than the nurse who knows it all. As a nurse, the opportunity to learn something new every day exists. Understanding this concept goes a long way in avoiding mistakes. Just about the time a nurse gains a certain comfort level with the job, thinking he or she has done or seen everything, something new will arise and it is back to square one. When this happens, it is like the first day on the job all over again. Confusion sets in, followed by urgency, and then the inevitable happens: a mistake is made.

It is not hard to recognize the nurse that knows it all. He or she is the nurse that makes comments such as, "I know how to use that machine, I don't need an in-service," or "they couldn't have changed it that much because it is the same brand." Arrogance leads to trouble, and that trouble is usually in the form of a mistake. No one knows everything about anything, and the best advice that one nurse can give another nurse is this: refreshers are never a bad thing. Don't be arrogant. Take time to learn the new technology and never make any assumptions about anything.

Arrogance doesn't solely lie within a nurse. Patients and their families can be guilty of knowing it all also. When discharging a patient, the nurse must go over discharge instructions including medications. Be leery of the family member that states, "mama's been on that medication for years, it's the little yellow pill." This can lead to a mistake if the nurse takes the family member's word for it and doesn't follow through on the discharge instructions. The doctor may have prescribed a new dosage, and in turn the pill will be a different color.

Also, it is a good idea to convey to the family members and the patient the need to throw away the old bottle of medication immediately and start with the new medication. There is a reason why the doctor changed the medication, and waiting until the old medication is completed is contraindicated in the patient's overall health plan. If either the patient or family member thinks that the aforementioned practice is acceptable, then being guilty of arrogance has occurred because either party is assuming more knowledge than the doctor. Never assume that the patient or the family members understand dosages, medications, or new instructions, make them repeat the instructions to ensure comprehension.

Arrogance is a tricky subject. Nurses need to learn how to best deal with the nuances involved in arrogance from four standpoints: themselves, coworkers, patients and their family members. Understanding that mistakes can result from arrogance is the first step in preventing these types of mistakes.

Intuition

As a new nurse, there is limited experience to draw from, but people in general have an innate sense or intuition about surroundings, people, and events. This comes from the survival instinct that was once utilized much more than today. Even though this instinct may be buried deep within one's psyche, it is still there. Today this instinct is partially recognized as intuition. Intuition is the ability to recognize clues or indicators that aren't readily tangible. Parts of intuition include: subtle clues of changes, a gut feeling that things just are not the way they should be, or something is out of place and doesn't fit. These are just a few examples of what can be classified as intuition. The following states some specific indicators of intuition that nurses need to be aware of.

Something that just isn't right could be as simple as a patient reaching for a glass of water and missing, or repeating the same question over and over without a history of doing so. Or, it could be a blank stare. These are all minor clues where intuition will come into play. If a nurse's gut tells them that something is wrong, then it usually is. Should you take this information to an experienced nurse? The answer is never cut and dry; sometimes the answer is yes and sometimes it is no. These types of instances are where sound judgment must come into play.

Time and experience will give the nurse the tools to deal with these types of "gut feelings", but in the meantime it is always best to error on the side of caution. Should you discuss the situation with the patient's family members? Always. Family members know the patient better than anyone else. The family can be a wealth of information. However, the family can also mislead a nurse when they are in denial about a patient's worsening condition. Do you alert the doctor? Do you wait a bit and come back for further evaluation? These are all viable options, and either way the nurse must have a plan to implement and follow through with the intuition factor. Never summarily dismiss intuition, as this would be a mistake.

An example of following one's intuition is as follows: suppose there is a restless patient and the doctor orders an IM injection for sedation. The nurse administers the drug, and the patient becomes sedate seven minutes later. The nurse finds this odd because the medication should have taken thirty minutes to work. Believing that something else is wrong, the nurse begins assessing the patient based on his or her intuition. During the assessment, the nurse checks the patient's pupils. The right pupil is larger than the left. This is a major problem. The reality is that the patient was restless due to a subarachnoid bleed. If the nurse would have ignored his or her intuition and been satisfied with the fact that the patient became sedate as ordered, then further investigation would not have happened. There is no way to know when the bleed would have been found. This type of mistake can cost a patient his or her life.

Ignoring one's intuition can cause a flurry of adverse effects. Take the time to seek out answers when something seems out of place or just not right. Realizing that intuition plays a key role in patient care can thwart mistakes and result in better overall care for the patient.

Assumption

"Assume" is a term that most people know the meaning of. The colloquial witticism of making an ass out of you and me is true, and a nurse should never assume anything. This is a huge mistake.

The simplest definition of assuming is the mistake of thinking that another person knows exactly what needs to be known. Another definition is not knowing what someone else doesn't know, but you think that they do know.

One example of assuming that is commonly taught in a BLS Healthcare provider CPR class is when someone yells for help and states, "Go get the AED." This is a communication error because the person needing help is not clear in the instructions and assumes that someone will help. If the person calls out indiscriminately and assumes that someone will go and get the AED, those people may make the assumption that someone else will go and get the AED. This endless cycle of assuming costs time, creates confusion, and the results can be fatal. The lesson behind this is to never assume. Be specific. Instead of just calling out to anyone, point at a specific person and say, "You in the pink shirt call 911 and get the AED." This avoids any chance of confusion and that person will know that they are the one that needs to go and get the AED instead of assuming that someone else will go.

Assumptions are dangerous during emergency situations. Nurses should speak up and state clearly the specific details about the situation. For instance, during a nurse's first code blue, the nurse should ensure that the team is aware of the fact that this is the first time working a cardiac arrest. If the new nurse is standing next to the code cart, the doctor or nurse will assume that the new nurse knows where the drugs and equipment are. This is due to the fact that the new nurse has situated him or herself in that role. The assumption made by the experienced physician or nurse will delay vital treatments in the process of trying to save a life. When in doubt, get out of the way. Also, when given an order that isn't understood tell the person immediately or else the assumption is made that the nurse understands.

For instance, in the trauma room the patient presents with a deviated trachea and absent breath sounds on the right. The experienced nurse and/or surgeon may assume that a nurse knows that this is a hemo/pneumothorax. When the doctor calls for a 30 French chest tube and the nurse fumbles through the drawers looking for the tube the patient's condition will worsen. This delay can cost a life. These types of instances can be prevented with communication, experience, and training. Avoiding the assumption process can deter many mistakes.

Communication

Communication errors are the most common types of mistakes that occur. Communication errors range from: reading orders, misunderstanding orders, cultural interpretations, non-verbal communications, face-to-face misunderstanding, and misinterpretations. A communication error is when one person tries to express an idea and the receiving party has an understanding that differs from the intended meaning.

An example of one type of communication error is classified as a cultural miscommunication. The following story illustrates one such instance. During a nursing shortage, several international nurses were hired. Culturally the relationships between the nurses and the physicians are vastly different as compared to the norm in the United States. The international nurses had no previous experience with PRN, or as needed, orders. Those nurses were accustomed to following orders as written and every medication has to be specifically spelled out. In their country, judgment wasn't allowed.

A week into orientation the realization of the cultural differences became apparent. Even though those nurses had the same license and passed the same test, it was evident that their educational backgrounds and communication styles were different. One such instance was during a conscious sedation procedure, the physician wrote for two PRN doses of versed and morphine.

After administering the first dose of each, the patient tolerated the procedure well. During cleanup, the student began drawing up the second doses of each medication. When asked what she was doing, the nurse stated, "I am following the physicians order. He wrote for two doses of versed and morphine." The patient was completely sedated and pain free with the initial doses and there was no need for the second doses. The international nurse had to be made aware of the meaning of PRN orders and that here, in the U.S., nurses are allowed to use their judgment in an instance such as this. This misunderstanding could have led to a potentially fatal situation.

In order to prevent communication errors, there needs to be clear and concise transference of information alongside the complete understanding of the idea being transferred. Due to multiple communication errors, the healthcare institution as a whole has implemented surgical and procedural timeouts, the limiting verbal orders, and using read-back and verified verbal orders, in order to close the loop in communication. These procedures are meant to eliminate the mistakes caused by communication errors.

Summary

This section is intended to educate nurses on the types of mistakes that can and do occur in the field of nursing. Even though the list isn't exhaustive, this is a good start for new nurses to begin learning about mistakes and ways to prevent the mistake from ever happening.

SECTION II: CLASSICATIONS OF MISTAKES

The previous section described the common errors leading up to reportable mistakes. The following section outlines and defines four classifications of patient related mistakes and the possible outcomes of each type.

Near misses

The classification of "near misses" is the least harmful of the four classifications covered in this section. The definition of a "near miss" is as follows: the patient was not in direct contact with the mistake. In other words, "near misses" are corrected prior to reaching the patient. One example of a near miss would be when the medication reconciliation record has been corrected with the right dose prior to the patient being discharged. Another example is when the pharmacy sends the wrong dose of a medication and the nurse recognizes the error prior to hanging or administering it. A near miss is when the potential for harm is present, but the mistake was caught and prevented from reaching the patient.

Just because the near miss never reached the patient doesn't mean it should ever be overlooked or underestimated. A nurse should report the near miss. This allows administration to identify the problem and use correct measures in order to prevent the mistake from being duplicated. This allows for the system error in the process to change. Nurses have to familiarize themselves with the institution's process and guidelines for reporting mistakes.

Mistakes That Reach the Patient Without Harm

The second classification of mistakes is the mistakes that reach the patient without harm. These types of mistakes are ones that physically reach the patient, such as the wrong antibiotic being administered, and are known as mistakes that reach the patient without harm. There are few things that are more heart breaking than looking up at an infusing antibiotic and seeing a different patient's name, antibiotic, or dose.

Once the mistake has been realized, there are policies and procedures that have to be followed. Such procedures may include actions such as: discontinuing the medication, notification of the mistake to the leadership team, and notifying the patient's physician.

These mistakes are often avoidable, but they do happen and nurses should do their best to prevent them. Even though these mistakes don't cause any physical harm, the potential for the harm exists and can lead to the next two classifications if not caught in time.

Mistakes That Reach the Patient With Harm

This classification is when a mistake has occurred in which physical reactions effect a patient's condition negatively, also known as harm. Patient outcomes can quickly proceed to this level when errors have occurred. When the mistake reaches the patient a physiological response is expected and can have consequences. Just as in the example listed above in the second classification, the incorrect antibiotic could lead to anaphylaxis. Then, further medical intervention is required to correct the mistake.

When these mistakes happen, quick thinking and actions are required. This is not the time to place blame. The patient's health is the priority. Treat the symptoms and then investigate the root cause at a later time. Ask for help from more experienced nurses, notify the physician, and continually assess the patient for deterioration and the response to the corrective action administered. The above-mentioned notification systems will be managed by notifying risk-management. Be sure that local protocols and procedures that are in place in the institution are followed, as there are no universal guidelines pertaining to this subject. Each place of employment will have its own set of rules in place, and knowing those rules is essential.

Catastrophic Mistakes

The fourth classification of a mistake is one that ends in catastrophe. This type of mistake is the worst-case scenario. Loss of limb or life is involved in catastrophic mistakes. One example of this would be when the patient mentioned above in the third classification has irreversible anaphylaxis and dies. This type of mistake has numerous adverse effects on the patient, his or her family, the nurse, and administration. When loss of life or limb occurs, the patient suffers the most. This in turn leads to life changing events for everyone involved. If the nurse or doctor is found at fault, lawsuits will ensue creating a ripple effect of devastation. These types of mistakes should be avoided at all costs.

SECTION III: PREVENTION
Prevention

The most important key to mistakes in healthcare is prevention. Nurses need to be aware of the most likely situations that make one vulnerable to committing an error. This type of education comes with experience, but it should be at the forefront of a nurse's mind everyday. Prevention, prevention, prevention; this statement cannot be stressed enough.

Nurses need to be aware of factors that influence mistakes such as:

- Do mistakes happen more often in the last 4 hours of a 12-hour shift?
- Is it omission of key data during an admission assessment?
- Are mistakes made due to lack of knowledge or arrogance?
- Is it a staffing issue?

A combination of any or all of these influences increases the likelihood of making a lethal mistake. Identifying the potential and risk factors involved in making mistakes will play a key roll in reducing the likelihood of the mistake ever occurring. Consider ways of avoiding these influences as a way to reduce the opportunity for mistakes to manifest. Remember the five Ps: "Prior Planning Prevents Poor Performance." Recognizing these potential situations aid nurses in developing a plan for prevention.

Be aware of high risk situations even when they happen often over the course of a typical shift, for instance: working in an emergency room and multiple trauma patients are being admitted back to back, new admissions at shift change, post-op recovery admitted at end of shift, being pulled to a new unit. These are just a few scenarios that impact the risk factor of mistakes. This is not an exhaustive list, but they are meant to be a few examples of the types of risks to identify because all of these things increase stress and diminish focus. During the workday and as experience is gained, nurses will learn to make mental notes of the types of risks that occur more often than not and ways to avoid them.

As stated in chapter four, one of the most important acts of prevention is checking the five Rs: right patient, right drug, right route, right dose, right time. Doing this every time will prevent medication errors. Not doing this can and will create a bad situation for all of those involved. The effects of a mistake can last a lifetime, and not only for the patient. The nurse that commits the error may never recover from the mistake either. The psychological impact can be overwhelming and can sometimes lead a nurse to choosing another career. More information about stress can be found in the next chapter.

Brian's Mistake

During my orientation to the ICU, the time came for me to administer medications on my own for the first time. In those days, nurses didn't have the luxury of pre-mixed medications. This meant going to the medication cabinet, getting the supplies on your own, and then mixing the medications.

It was time for one of my patient's noon antibiotic. The order read 500mg of Ceftizoxime. Due to my newness and not understanding the importance of paying close attention to details, I pulled out a vial of Cefixifime. I like to think that new nurses have it easier these days due to the mistakes I made early on in my career. This helps me placate my ego.

Anyway, I mixed the antibiotic by inserting the 20 gauge disposable straight needle into the infusion port hub and injecting the med into the usual 100cc bag of normal saline. Next, I spiked the bag with the tubing. Then, after calculating my drip rate to infuse over one hour, I used the roller clamp to set the drip.

After completing this task, my preceptor entered the patient's room, and boomed, "When did the Doctor change antibiotics?"

"Ah, ah, he didn't." I stammered.

"I hope this label is wrong! It's not the antibiotic that's ordered," she continued.

"Wh, Wh, What do you mean?" I mumbled.

My first medication error had been discovered, and on my very first try nonetheless. Thoughts of panic began racing through my head, "Where did I fail? Was it my arrogance, stupidity, lack of knowledge or the pharmacy companies for having such close spellings?"

The next two hours of the day were grueling punishment. In no particular order, I spent the time calling the doctor, researching the adverse interactions, notifying the family, writing an incident report, and fearing for my job and this man's life.

During my research everything I read contained the word "anaphylaxis." My patient is going to die, I just knew it. Luckily the patient survived without any harm, but my first mistake left a lasting impression. Thirty years later, I triple check my medication labels before administering any medications.

-6-

Emotions

"A cheerful heart is good medicine, but a crushed spirit dries up the bones."

-Proverbs 17:22

Introduction

Death is a natural part of life. It is unavoidable. As of yet, there has been no known record of anyone escaping this inevitability. Death is the exact opposite of what nurses and healthcare professionals everywhere stand for. The Hippocratic Oath states that medical professionals should "pursue lifelong learning to better care for the sick and to prevent illness." Death destroys this ideal; it is the nemesis of the prevention of sickness and illness. No one can change the fact that people die, but learning how to deal with death when it happens is a huge part of being a nurse.

It is only natural to get emotionally attached to patients, especially patients that resemble family or friends. One such example would be an elderly man that reminds the nurse of his or her grandfather. The feelings for the grandfather may manifest toward the patient in the same manner. When this happens, the patient becomes the real grandfather and the emotional attachment is then the same. The patient lying in the bed is viewed as a relative instead of a person that they do not know. This is where an underlying issue can develop. It is one thing to show compassion and caring for a patient, but it is another when emotions interfere with patient care due to clouded judgment. Getting emotionally attached to a patient can lead to compassionate choices rather than the science of caring and healing. Awareness of such a situation is pertinent. Professionalism must be maintained at all times, and one way to ensure that professionalism is maintained is to treat every patient with the same amount of care and compassion. Regardless of emotional ties that stem from looks, attitudes, suffering, or longevity of the patient encounter, every patient is due the same amount of objectivity and care.

Stress

When seconds count and precision matters there are no room for errors. This kind of pressure from high stakes situations coupled with the knowledge that life or death events can happen at any given moment is enough to cause anyone to become emotionally charged. It is hard for most people to watch as others around them suffer. Compassion is a natural feeling. Creating bonds with patients is also a side effect of the job. This can happen in a matter of minutes or can take several days. Either way, once a connection has been made and a nurse becomes emotionally invested in a patient it creates a certain amount of stress on the nurse. Some nurses may handle that stress well while others do not. Furthermore, this stress may manifest at any time and nurses are prone to break down at any given moment when the stress level becomes too much to handle.

There are numerous ways to handle the stress, and people often handle stress differently because there is not just one way to handle stress. Sometimes, the process requires some experimentation in order to figure out the way that works best for a particular individual. Most people handle stress in their own way and at their own pace. Try the four "A's" for dealing with stress:

1.   Acceptance: some things are simply beyond one's control and cannot be changed. A firm realization of the situation is the first step in finding a way to deal with the stress inducer. Finding a way to deal with the stress is easier once the person realizes that there is no way to "fix" the problem. In turn, the situation has to be made tolerable not "fixed."

2.   Attitude: one person's emergency is not necessarily another person's emergency. Perception of the situation can go a long way in finding the "silver lining" in a less than favorable occurrence. Having a "can do" attitude versus a "doom and gloom" attitude can make a world of difference. Focus on the positive and don't get bogged down with the negatives. Attitude is everything. If one chooses to find the good in things, the bad doesn't seem to be so bad.

3.   Avoidance: Take a look at the big picture by asking the question, "Will this matter next week, what about next month? Will anybody even remember this situation ever happened? If not, then there is no reason to get weighed down by the problem in the first place. Walk away from the situation and never look back. Never discount the act of doing nothing. Avoiding the situation is sometimes the best course of action. If the problem is not worth the time, then don't spend any time on it. Don't make problems bigger than they need to be. Take a deep breath and move on.

4.   Appeasement: Take care of yourself first. Find something that helps you relax and do that thing often, daily if possible. Take some time to unwind all knots that have been tied over the course of the day or the week. These knots don't just disappear on their own; they just keep piling up and making a mess of one's nerves. Make a concerted effort to relax and enjoy something. Appease yourself and then you are ready to help someone else. (This topic is covered in depth in Chapter 8).

Crying

One thing nurses should know is the fact that crying is ok. Crying is a natural process and is part of dealing with sad situations. Don't believe anyone that says otherwise. Some nurses may see crying as being unprofessional in front of patients, while other nurses may say that it is ok to cry with their patients. In the end, it depends on the individual nurse and the situation.

As with anything, planning is a must. If a nurse stays in the business long enough the urge to cry will happen. Nurses should expect this and be proactive in formulating a plan for when the inevitable happens. A well thought out plan is being proactive versus the alternative of being reactive and caught in a potentially bad situation. Nurses should understand that eventually their emotions will get the better of them and should be prepared for such an occasion. One good idea is to find a refuge within the hospital to go and take a break. Having a quiet place to sort out one's thoughts is essential. Even in the most intense situations nurses understand the dynamics involved in patient care and the emotions that are associated with such practices. Find a way to take a breather, get away from the emotional baggage, and compose one's self. There is nothing wrong with this practice and it allows the nurse to regroup and continue on with the job.

Another helpful idea is to have someone reliable to share with when bad situations occur. A clergyman, another nurse, or a mentor are all valid choices. Family members should be held in reserve as in many situations they just don't understand the stress and details associated with the situation enough to help. It is easier to find help and support from people who share in the same types of situations that cause one to grieve. The key to success in this situation is planning. Don't wait until the situation presents itself; find a support person early on.

In many cases, the hospital offers grief counselors for staff as well as patients and family members. These people are trained professionals and are always a good choice for dealing with strife. Inquire about such services during orientation. The service is provided for a reason and there is no shame in using these services where offered. A nurse should never be afraid to ask for help.

Yelling

Yelling is an unfortunate part of nursing. Doctors yell, patients yell, patient's family members yell, and nurses yell at each other. Nursing is an emotionally charged work environment. Yelling is a part of the job. It is important for new nurses to understand that raised voices are not uncommon. But why?

Where life and death is concerned, emotions run high. Handling one's emotions sometimes end in an anger response—shouting. The person shouting often times feels trapped and frustrated and doesn't know what else to do. So, in turn, yelling ensues. This emotional response really doesn't accomplish anything other than gaining attention. Remember this point, when people shout they are trying to get someone's attention.

This type of behavior is a learned response, and some people exercise the response more than others. In the end, yelling is a response to a situation that has frustrated the speaker and that person wants to get the attention of his or her audience. The natural response to being shouted at is to shout back. This is not the correct response. Two wrongs do not make a right. Take the higher ground and try to get to the root of the problem instead of getting caught up in the emotional response of the person that is frustrated. Practicing good psychology is a key element in dealing with someone who is yelling. There are three natural responses that people have when they are being yelled at. They are fight, flight, or freeze. Unfortunately, none of these are the proper response as far as nurses are concerned.

Nurses should avoid fighting at all cost. This is often the type of response that the initiator is searching for, hence the term "picking a fight." Fighting is never a professional response and should be avoided at all costs. Avoiding a fight demonstrates self-control and professionalism and will lead to an acceptable outcome.

Flight is an acceptable response, but running away from a problem is not because the problem has not been resolved. Just remember not to fly too far because the natural instinct for a predator is to give chase. Fleeing in this type of situation means to remove one's self from the volatile situation until the other party has had some time to calm down. It does not mean to avoid the situation until shift change because the problem then becomes the next nurse's problem. This is often times easier said than done, but an attempt to remove one's self from the situation should be the first course of action. Having someone chase another person down a hallway yelling draws a great deal of attention, and that just feeds into the problem and does not provide a resolution. If this happens, the person should stop and face the accuser. If removing one's self from the situation is not possible then the person being yelled at should keep calm and look for a reasonable resolution.

Freezing is not advised, as this allows the initiator the opportunity to gain the upper hand as they detect fear. Whether or not the person being shouted at is afraid or not is irrelevant. It is the perception of fear given by the act of freezing that gives way to the notion. The correct way to handle a volatile situation is to be an active participant in the conversation while keeping a calm and even tone in his or her voice when speaking. The frustrated person will eventually tire of yelling and the fact that a rational response is reciprocated instead of an emotional response will send the message that the respondent is in control.

In summary, remain in control of one's emotions, always be an active listener, and be a rational respondent instead of emotional one. The main point offered in the above information is that situations of intense emotions exist in the field of nursing and that yelling happens.

The following story illustrates the stress that nurses will face while on the job. Gloria was in her first year on the job in the emergency room of a small community hospital when she witnessed her first case of child abuse.

Gloria's Nightmare

The overhead intercom rang out, "Five-minute ETA. Three year old severe burns trauma room." I didn't know how to feel, I was excited when I first got assigned to be part of the trauma team, but knowing that I actually had to work on a child with burns, my stomach rumbled as I fought back the nausea.

The doors flung open, and the stretcher flew into the hall. The paramedics burst through the treatment room doors with a crying, semi-limp, badly burned three year old with singed, malodorous golden blond hair the same color of my own child's. The doctor started spouting out orders and the other nurses crowded around the child and started working. The room quickly got crowded, so I took it upon myself to start the chart. I perched myself behind the rolling chart cart. Pen in hand, I scribbled notes as fast as the doctor was giving orders.

During the flourish of activity, I looked around and saw my brother standing just outside the door frozen with a look of terror on his face. My mind raced, "what is he doing here?" I looked back toward the hospital bed. Through the sea of people I caught a glimpse of the child's face; it was my niece. My heart jumped up into my throat as my knees buckled and I grabbed for the cart for support.

"Gloria," a voice yelled repeatedly, "Gloria, what the hell is wrong with you? Call for a helicopter, we need to get this child to the burn unit." I heard the voices, but I couldn't move. I was too weak to move or even respond. "You need to move," the charge nurse screamed at me with her face directly in front of mine. Tears welled up in my eyes, and I broke down. The tears were flowing, I began screaming frantically at the doctor and at the other nurses. Security was just outside the room, at the direction of the charge nurse, I was removed.

I was taken to the family counseling room, as I sat there crying endlessly security showed up again. This time they were escorting my brother, the social worker, and a police officer. There was a moment of silence just before the barrage of questions started flowing from the social worker. During the questioning, I overheard way more information than I was prepared to handle.

My brother had left my niece alone with his girlfriend when he went off to play basketball with his friends. He was gone about four hours before returning home to find his child lying on the bathroom floor with multiple burns all over her body. When he found her huddled on the floor, he noticed that the curling iron was still plugged in and still on. When my brother told this to the social worker I lost it and started beating on him. I attacked my brother and had to be restrained and forcibly removed from the room.

I was escorted to a separate family counseling room where a security guard was posted in order to assure that I would not leave the room. A little while later, a chaplain from the hospital arrived in my room and tried to diffuse my anger. I don't really recall much of the conversation as I have tried to block most of the psychological trauma from my memory. But what I do remember from those events are not pleasant ones. As it turns out, she had taken the hot iron and repeatedly burned my niece for a total of 31 times. This woman had babysat my own child on more than one occasion. I could not believe that one person could be capable of this type of torture on an innocent child. It was just too much for me to process.

Looking back, I probably could have handled the situation differently, but the whole ordeal was too much for me. I just couldn't handle that kind of stress. Luckily, the hospital was kind enough only to suspend me for a short period of time while I attended grief-counseling sessions. Upon my return to work, I had been transferred out of the emergency department and was assigned to a floor in the hospital. The official reason for the transfer was a suspicion that I could not handle the stress and the hospital administration feared that another child abuse case would adversely affect me in the future. I was made aware of the fact that the only reason they were willing to work with me and allow me to keep my job at the hospital after the incident was due to the fact that this involved a family member.

Ten years later, I realize that I have faced the most dreaded situation that a nurse can be exposed to—working on a family member. For me this nightmare was a reality.

Summary
This chapter covers the topic of emotions and offers some insight on how nurses can deal with

them. Stress is an unavoidable force that occurs in the field of nursing. Recognizing stress and formulating ways to deal with the stress is as important as breathing. Stress must be dealt with and formulating a plan is a good way to deal with the inevitable. Crying is a natural part of the job. When the stakes are life or death, it is virtually impossible not to have an emotional involvement. Finding a good place to cry, meditate, or reflect is an important way to deal with this stressor. Yelling happens, and it is important for a nurse to understand this dynamic and find a proper way to handle those volatile situations. The story in this chapter reflects an actual situation in which crying and yelling were both factors that lead to unbearable stress and the eventual emotional downfall of a practicing nurse. Gloria's worst nightmare had come true.

-7-

You

"Nurses are a unique kind. They have this insatiable need to care for others, which is both their biggest strength and fatal flaw."
-Dr. Jean Watson

Introduction

In a service-oriented society, the customer always comes first. The healthcare field is no exception. The customer in this particular instance is the patient, and one must also remember that in this particular field the customer is not always right. The hard part is maintaining one's dignity in spite of that fact. Think about it, if patients were always right then there would be no need for medical professionals to exist. However, one has to be realistic about the situation and the goals that are expected of nurses. Putting the patient at the top of your to-do-list is very important, but new nurses must learn to take this idea one step further in practice. There are very few careers in the world that have more stress in them than nursing does. With this in mind, nurses need to learn how to take care of themselves first, and then they can start to take care of their patients.

If a nurse is distracted, the patient will suffer. Who benefits in a situation such as this? The obvious answer is no one. This is the moment when things can turn very bad very quickly. Any outside distractions that are keeping the nurse's head out of the game can and will eventually lead to disaster. In order to maintain the high level of professionalism that is expected, a nurse must be able to separate work related issues from home life issues and stay focused on the task at hand. Focus is important for a nurse as it relates to success.

The issue at hand is the fact that expectations do not change just because the nurse is having a bad day, and why should they? Can the fact that one's teenage son ran up an enormous cell phone bill by purchasing apps for the phone really compare to the problem that your patient is facing—liver failure? If the cell phone issue clouds the mind instead of focusing on giving the patient with the failing liver the absolute best possible care then two wrongs have occurred. First, the nurse isn't doing the job, and the second part is the fact that the patient has suffered because of the neglect. One key to survival in being a nurse is keeping your sanity and staying healthy. Outlined below are some different steps that can be taken to achieve homeostasis.

Sleep

An important part of any healthy lifestyle is to get plenty of rest. When tired—sleep. It is ok to take a nap on days off. Don't get caught up in the fact that hundreds of things need to be done. If you're too tired to do them then you are not doing yourself or anyone else any favors by pushing through the tiredness to get these things done. Just like when at work, a nurse must learn to prioritize. The same applies for home life;

prioritize and then attack, but be well rested in the meantime.

According to the Mayo Clinic website, adults require seven to nine hours of quality sleep a night. Noted sleep expert Dr. Morgenthaler states, "If your sleep is frequently interrupted or cut short, you're not getting quality sleep — and the quality of your sleep is just as important as the quantity." Quality sleep can be achieved in many different ways. One way is to make sure your room is dark, especially when working the night shift. Some good solutions are to choose a darker color paint for the walls and utilize room darkening shades, blinds, and curtains to block out the sunlight that comes through windows and doors. Also, keep the telephone out of the bedroom unless expecting a call. Find another way of being contacted if at all possible while sleeping. There are few things worse than being awakened by a telephone call from someone who wants to sell something. Ask a neighbor to be an emergency contact or work out another system with family for dealing with these kinds of situations and emergencies.

Make sure to have a comfortable bed. After all, people spend one-third of their lives in bed so why not make the best of it. Also, think about using a white noise machine. The soothing sounds have been proven to induce a fuller and deeper sleep.

Being well rested helps every aspect of your life. Morgenthaler claims, "Although some people claim to feel rested on just a few hours of sleep a night, research shows that people who sleep so little over many nights don't perform as well on complex mental tasks as do people who get closer to seven hours of sleep a night." This claim directly relates to nurses, and nurses should make sure that they get enough sleep to complete numerous complex mental tasks. Sleep is important, don't neglect it.

Eating

Eat well. Don't skip meals. After all, food is how the human body gains energy. A well-rounded diet is important. Eating healthy should be a priority. Don't be tempted by what is fast and easy due to a hectic work life. However, going into the job with the mindset of eating healthy will eventually become second nature. Later on, these healthy choices will pay off.

Skipping meals while at work is not good; while this may often times be unavoidable, nurses should make sure that if and when they snack that they are making smart food choices. Don't be tempted and lured in by coworkers bad habits and the endless supply of cookies in the break room. Get into the mindset of eating healthy and avoid missing meals. Nursing is an active job and energy is essential. Be sure to "eat right."

Volunteering

Being a nurse is stressful. This fact is unavoidable. However, there are ways to deal with stress. One way is to volunteer. It is acceptable and encouraged to put nursing skills and abilities to work in a fun way. There are many opportunities for nurses to volunteer such as: manning a first-aid station at charity events, summer camps, marathons, walkathons, or even teaching first-aid.

Volunteering has a two-fold result. First, it gives a self-esteem boost. Everyone likes to be appreciated and by volunteering one can gain respect and are often praised for the effort. Second, it helps the community. Often times there is a need for specialized volunteers at events and social gatherings that would otherwise be a cost to the hosting organization. Volunteering as a nurse and putting nursing skills to use in order to serve the community saves money and fills a need. Civic duty is not a requirement, but helping others on a volunteer basis is a win-win scenario. Choose an organization that is a good fit, and then help out when needed.

Alone Time

Everyone needs some alone time. Time to kick back, relax, and do the things that are enjoyable. Like reading a book, going for a walk, or playing with a pet. Find time to do something enjoyable that is relaxing and unwind. Being a nurse is stressful and the job can overwhelm a person if a way to deal with the stress is not utilized. Finding a coping mechanism is important. There are many things a nurse can do for themselves that make them feel good.

This shouldn't be viewed as narcissistic behavior; instead, it should be viewed as a type of therapy. Everyone needs a momentary escape from the daily grind in which to unravel the big ball of stress that has been rolling up both on the job and off the clock. This kind of action can be referred to as the "care for one's self." Nurses spend a great deal of time caring for others. It is easy to fall into the trap of forgetting to care for one's self.

Find a way to get away from repetitive activities, even if only for a moment or two. The important thing to remember is that sometimes a person just needs some peace and quiet. Find a hobby, keep a journal, do some gardening, or just take a nap; it doesn't matter what the activity is as long as it focuses on the person doing it and no one else. That is why they call it "you" time.

This time should be spent on you, and no one else.

Working Too Much

A nurse is usually overworked on a daily basis. It is not uncommon to have more patients than what is considered to be a normal workload. There are many reasons behind this issue. One reason is the fact that people get tired, sick, or burnt out, and then that person doesn't show up for work. Another reason is the fact that hospitals are usually understaffed from the get go, not to mention the fact that there is still a deficit of nurses in the workforce altogether. People quit, get new jobs, get new careers, retire or get promoted and this also contributes to the staffing shortages.

All of the above reasons lead to the fact that hospitals offer massive amounts of overtime. Overtime is great, but there is only one aspect of overtime that is good—the money. On average nurses make a decent wage, but when overtime is calculated nurses can make a bundle of money. This is very tempting and lucrative to one's pocket book. However, this temptation can and will get the best of nurses if they are not adequately prepared.

The stress of the normal nurse's job is hard enough to deal with on a daily basis, but when compounded by a thirty-three percent increase in a person's work life the stress can get the best of anyone. If normal shifts are three twelve hour days or nights a week, working an extra shift increases the workweek by thirty-three percent. By many standards, it is hard to deny that the money is good, but all of the extra factors that are associated with working more are not good. It doesn't take long for all those extra factors to build up an insurmountable stress level, which can lead to burnout.

New nurses are cautioned against working too much. Administrators and supervisors will beg, plead, and praise those who are willing to work extra shifts. However, a nurse should remember that this is good for the business, but excess work will take its toll on a nurse's mental and physical health. Don't be afraid to say no. If extra work is wanted then work extra, but unless extra work is truly wanted, don't work. Remember, if a nurse can't take care of him or herself, then others can't be cared for. The following story is an example that illustrates the pitfalls of being overworked.

Jenny's Tragedy

Jenny works in a very busy emergency room. She is single and lives alone. Jenny has been on the job about nine months and is excelling at her job and has found a rhythm to her work, and she has been praised repeatedly for her efforts and what a good job she has been doing. She works the night shift for twelve hours from 7 p.m. to 7 a.m. She is new and because of it she has been assigned to work Thursday, Friday, and Saturday nights. This a not a great schedule for a young and single person, but Jenny doesn't mind because she gets night and weekend shift differentials and she really enjoys the money which helps to pay off her college loans.

Everything in Jenny's mind was proceeding to plan and she was gradually meeting the goals she had set for herself. She got a job in a busy ER and was being paid well. She had learned most of the protocols and procedures for her department and was executing things flawlessly at work. However, one day she made a mistake. The mistake almost cost a woman her life.

Jenny showed up to work on Thursday night at 6:15 pm, early as usual. The shift was busy. By the end of the shift, Jenny's relief had not shown up and she agreed to stay an extra two hours over to cover the patient load because the nurse that was supposed to be there was having car trouble and was going to be late. The nurse arrived around 8:45 a.m., and after giving the relief nurse reports on the patients that Jenny had been assigned, Jenny clocked out and headed home. Jenny has a thirty-five minute commute from her job to her apartment. After getting a hot shower and a quick bite to eat, Jenny laid down to sleep at around 11 a.m. She tossed and turned for a while and finally fell asleep and slept until 5 p.m. She dragged herself out of bed and was on the road by 5:30 p.m. She was always mindful of leaving herself plenty of time to get to work, and today was no different. She had accounted for traffic and showed up to work around her normal time.

Once again the ER was full, and Jenny had her hands full all shift. She managed one fifteen-minute break that enabled her to scarf down a sandwich she had bought from the vending machine. Thirty minutes before the end of the shift, the charge nurse announced that a cardiac patient was on the way to the ER and would be arriving by ambulance in about ten minutes. The patient was suffering from refractory ventricular tachycardia and had been cardioverted twice by the paramedics. The patient was hypotensive and in and out of consciousness. The charge nurse asked Jenny if she would mind helping out for a while until the patient was stable. Jenny did not hesitate to volunteer. Even though she was tired, Jenny was excited to have the opportunity to help out in this critical situation. It was a learning opportunity and she was not going to miss out on it.

After an hour of working, numerous interventions and drug therapies, the patient stabilized enough to be transferred to the

Intensive Care Unit. After transferring the patient to the unit, Jenny clocked out and headed home. When Jenny made it home she went straight to bed. Around 3 p.m. that Saturday afternoon Jenny's cell phone rang. It was the charge nurse. She explained to Jenny that one of the nurses had gotten a blood exposure and had to be taken off the floor of the department per protocol. This incident left them short-handed and the charge nurse asked Jenny if she would mind coming in early. Jenny had a problem turning down overtime and was always willing to help out in a pinch. So, Jenny agreed. After a quick shower, she went in to work. The shift was brutal. A constant influx of patients kept the entire emergency room busy all night.

After working fourteen hours straight, Jenny made her way out to her car and headed home. On the way home, Jenny called her mother using her cell phone. She recalls telling her mother how tired she was and how she had planned on sleeping the whole day and probably wasn't going to make it over to supper that night as they had planned. After hanging up, Jenny doesn't recall anything up until the point where she was violently woke up and her head felt as if it had just been hit with a sledgehammer. She couldn't focus, she had no idea what was happening, and then everything went blank again.

Jenny woke up several hours later only to find out she was lying in a hospital bed with her family hovering around her. After a bit of confusion, Jenny asked what had happened and why was she here. Jenny's father leaned over and told her that she was in a car wreck. She tried hard to remember, but she couldn't recall any details about the event. She asked her father again about what happened. He wasn't sure about telling her the details, as he was afraid that she wasn't ready to hear about the accident. Jenny pressed him further so eventually he gave in and told her that apparently—according to witnesses—she had fallen asleep, run through a red light, and had struck another car in the side.

The lady Jenny had struck suffered severe traumatic injuries and was unconscious and in the Intensive Care Unit at the time. After finding out the details about the other party involved, Jenny had only one thought, "It's all my fault."

Jenny's Conclusion

The above story illustrates how tragedy can occur from being too tired to focus. There is know way to prove that this event could have been prevented if Jenny wasn't too tired to drive, but it does make a compelling argument about the risks of working too much.

Home Life

There is an old saying that states "Don't bring your work home with you." In a nurse's case, it would be awkward to bring a patient home. However, in this instance the reverse is true. A nurse should not bring his or her home life to work. If a nurse is preoccupied by affairs at home, then he or she tends to not focus on the job and tasks at hand. The ability to separate the two, work life and home life, is instrumental in having a successful career and avoiding early burnout. Burnout happens when employees are consistently faced with high job demands, stressful working environments, and few resources to complete the job. Most burned-out nurses experience high levels of exhaustion, and they display negative attitudes about the job. The following story illustrates the importance of separating home life from work life and vice versa. Robin comes to this conclusion one day after work while talking with her husband.

Robin's Dilemma

Taking "patients" home after work isn't recommended. The reality for me is some are too emotionally charged not to. Not physically of course, but mentally. I recall one night in particular, it was the night I cared for a young trauma patient.

The night had started as routine as a 20 bed Trauma ICU could start. Then, the emergency room called. The person on the other end of the line wanted a bed for a multiple system trauma neurological patient. The charge nurse started to grumble, "Why are we getting another Neuro patient? The Neuro ICU has beds." Since I had a light assignment at the time, I volunteered for the admission. I quickly transferred my gunshot wound to the leg patient over to the step-down unit. Then, I prepared the bed for the incoming trauma patient by placing double padding for the blood loss and other bodily fluids that were going to be present.

I had just finished when the trauma team came rolling through the doors. One guy was bagging the patient, while another was yelling, "Is the ventilator set up?" Impersonating a flight deck controller, I motioned for the team to "land" the patient in the bed space. I quickly did a total body scan of the patient, and something just didn't look right. It wasn't the misaligned lower extremities with open fractures, nor the bulky blood soaked gauze bandage protruding from his abdomen. Instead, it was the fact that each time the chief trauma resident squeezed the BVM (bag-valve-mask) something was coming out of the side of the patient's head. "That's just not right," I thought to myself.

As the admitting nurse, it was my responsibility to take control of the airway; so, I did. Overall, it was a smooth hand off from the trauma resident to the ICU team. The transfer of care report started without the respiratory therapist or a ventilator present. I was still bagging the patient, and my eyes were focused on the side of the patient's head.

The chief resident began spouting out a litany of traumatic injuries, one of which was an open occipital fracture. Every time I squeezed the bag the mess on the bed grew larger. My curiosity got the best of me. Pointing at the side of the patient's head, I asked, "What's this?"

"That's his brains coming out, I gotta go wash my hands," the chief resident replied. The tissue and blood had worked its way up the chief's forearms, half way to his elbows.

The specialty teams began to arrive. Orthopedics was first; the team worked flawlessly splinting and dressing the numerous fractures on both lower and upper extremities preparing the patient for surgery. Next, the cardio thoracic surgery team prepped and inserted bilateral chest tubes. The neuro-surgery team was the last to arrive. It was now time to look at what had been haunting and intriguing me from the start. We log rolled the patient, and then the C-Collar was removed for access to the occipital injury. During the course of the assessment, I watched as the surgeon inspected the avulsed scalp tissue. It had some bone fragments and grey matter in it. The surgeon looked up at me and said, "It only matters if it's grey matter."

They rushed the patient from the room straight to surgery. I was done with my portion of the trauma alert, and the patient had made it to the operating room. It was my turn to go wash up. I scrubbed for what seemed to be an eternity. I finished just in time for shift change.

Leaving work, I was emotionally and physically spent. On the ride home I had picked up an emotional "hitch hiker". I couldn't stop thinking about that trauma patient.

I arrived home just as my husband was getting ready to leave for work. We were standing in the kitchen chatting. My spouse asked, "How was your night?"

There was a pause as I was trying to figure out a way to summarize the shift. How do I explain the horrific night I had just had to my husband? He is an information technologist, but will he really understand?

I started gushing out details and information. I should have noticed the multiple attempts to change the subject, the defensive body language, fidgeting hands and feet. I continued my emotional purge right there in the kitchen.

Suddenly my husband spoke up and said, "If you don't like your job just quit!" This statement jolted me back into reality. I shut up, kissed him goodnight, and headed for bed.

It was right then that I realized what bringing my work home meant. How could my family understand what I do for a living, and for that matter, can anyone other than another nurse ever really understand?

Main Points

Having a healthy home life is important. Your personal time should be yours; use it wisely. Take care of yourself and take care of your family. It's hard to care for those closest to you when all you do every day at work is take care of others. Don't neglect the needs of yourself, your family, and your friends.

When striving to be the best, first take certain steps in order to make sure of being in the right mindset for taking care of yourself, taking care of patients, and taking care of the family. Things that will help are: turning down overtime (unless truly wanted), treating yourself to something relaxing and fun, and proper eating and sleeping habits. Talking things out are an important part of dealing with stress. Find a mentor, clergy, counselor, or just a friend with whom you can vent. A nurse must find a way of handling the stress of the job. One key aspect of surviving the

job of being a nurse is the ability to take care of
one's self.

-8-

Seriously

"We may not be able to change the world, but we can laugh at it. Sometimes that's enough. It's good to remember that when we hear patients laughing, we're hearing the sounds of their bravery. "

-Karen Buxman

Introduction

One of the best assets a nurse can have is the ability to laugh at one's self. The job of healing is deeply rooted in tradition, and is serious business. While this is true, it doesn't mean a nurse cannot laugh. There is an old proverb that claims that laughter is the best medicine. In many cases this is true. However, there is another way to approach the seriousness of the job. Do so with a smile on your face and a flame of passion in your heart. Happiness is contagious. This concept may not be an easy one to understand, but once a nurse understands the underlying message presented in the following pages hopefully they will profit from the knowledge that laughter can help in the healing process.

Perfection

Nurses are required to be experts in medicine and practical skills, and to stay abreast of cutting edge technology. This isn't an easy task. Also, nurses are required to be the eyes and ears of the doctor. Nurses need to provide care for the sick in ways that cannot readily be defined, and definitions concerning nursing are in a constant state of flux. Nurses have to be comfortable in the most serious of situations, and perform flawlessly in an instant. Nurses are expected to be perfect even when the rules are constantly changing and emotions dictate actions rather than logic or acceptable practices. Nurses are expected to know human physiology alongside human psychology, and they must do so expeditiously.

One can very easily make the claim that the very idea of these aforementioned notions is absurd. No one is flawless. Human beings are complicated, and every individual is unique within his or her own right. It is this uniqueness that is often times overlooked in the medical profession. There are no two people are exactly the same, and until cloning becomes a widespread accepted practice two people will never be the same. So how can a nurse be expected to be perfect when no one else can? Well, they can't. However, with the proper skills, mentality, and insight into human nature nurses can do their jobs, do them well, and offer hope as well as healthcare to a patient.

Relationships

Medicine is a serious business and is probably one of the most confusing and mysterious aspects of the human experience. The only other thing that even comes close to being this complicated is human relationships, which of course is a part of nursing. Every human body is unique, and so is the mind. No two people think exactly the same way. Scholars have been trying for centuries to classify and catalogue the human mind. They try to understand the how and why behind the decisions that are made based on emotions rather than logic. Psychologists have been trying to fit round pegs into square holes, and no matter how hard they try the two just don't go together. They want everything to fit nicely into a box, and unfortunately the mind just doesn't work that way. Often times, theorists alongside medical professionals feel that there should be only one right answer, and some of them spend their entire lives in pursuit of that answer. Sometimes, people try so hard to prove a theory that they often forget what the problem was in the first place. This type of mentality can be detrimental in the science of healing.

How does all of this relate to being a nurse? Well, there is no right answer to this question. That is exactly the point. More times than not, there isn't a right answer. People do not fit into molds. Everyone is different, and when a nurse understands and embraces the idea of diversity, the easier it will be for him or her to build relationships with patients.

Healthcare is much more than diagnosis, pills, or surgery. The human being is made up of mind, body, and spirit. It is these three things that must be cared for during the healing process. It is this knowledge that can make or break a nurse. If a nurse treats the patient as a whole, addressing the mind, body, and spirit, then the patient will better respond to the care provided. If a nurse ignores these things the situation becomes problematic and complicated.

Caring for the patient inevitably includes building a relationship with him or her. It is the give and take, the compromises, the understanding, and expectations of roles and how a nurse interacts with the patient that builds relationships. Why are relationships important? Simply stated—trust. If a patient does not trust the nurse, then there is a break down in the process. How does one build trust? Honesty, integrity, genuineness, and the ability to be perceived as a human rather than an uncaring robot are things that contribute to building trust between a nurse and a patient.

Patient Care

No matter how much science encroaches into the job of being a nurse, no matter how much administration pressures nurses to be robots, no matter how indifferent society is about proper healthcare, the stark reality is that patient care should be the main focus of a nurse. Care is a complicated issue and can be defined in many ways, but nurses are expected to provide care despite the various definitions of it. Tradition dictates that nurses are nurturers. Nurturing is caring. Research has concluded that nursing is considered to be a "mothering act." Regardless of gender, nurses are expected to be a mother hen that hovers over her young, protects them from harm, and sees to their needs until they are able to fend for themselves. This analogy represents the expectations from the patient's point of view as well as what is accepted practice in the field of nursing. The patient expects nurses to care about them and to care for them. That is the job of a nurse.

The robot stereotype is often used in healthcare to describe a caregiver that is cold, callous, and uncaring. It is often times the nurse or doctor that practices from a science perspective rather than a holistic practice that gets this label. Traditionally, this was called bedside manner, but it is slowly being replaced with the robot stereotype—also known as artificial intelligence. With the advent of the Internet, anyone can claim to be an "expert." With information so readily available, it only takes a Smartphone and an Internet connection to verify facts. Nurses must now keep this fact in the back of their minds. It is easy to verify information, and suspicious statements can easily be researched.

Verifying information given to the patient by a nurse is another avenue that patients can use to prove the trustworthiness of a nurse. Do not ever give a patient a reason to be suspicious. Speak the truth, and give information in terms that the patient understands. Misunderstanding causes tension, anxiety, and sense of low self-esteem. These three things are counterproductive in the process of healing. Nurses should avoid creating such instances in a consistent manner. There are many ways a nurse can ease tension, and being honest is one of the best ways to gain trust and begin building relationships with patients.

Laughter

One good way to put a patient at ease is to make them laugh. Other ways are: do not be critical of the patient, do not judge a person concerning the current situation, and keep the patient's feelings in mind. If the opportunity presents itself to make light of the situation, then the nurse should take advantage of the moment. If the patient sees the nurse not taking the situation too seriously, the patient becomes more comfortable with what is going on concerning the current problem. For instance, if a nurse detects that the patient becomes anxious just before the administration of an injection, an opportunity exists there to use laughter in calming the patient.

A nurse could use an approach like this: "I can't lie. This is going to hurt, but only for a second. Think of it like a bee sting, and those little suckers die after they sting you." If the patient doesn't laugh then go get the topical numbing solution. Taking the extra time to prove that the nurse cares, and that he or she is willing to do anything to make the shot as painless as possible will prove to the patient that the nurse really does care. Even though the fact exists that no matter how hard one tries, no one can please everyone all the time, but that shouldn't dissuade the nurse from trying.

The following is a story concerning a nurse named Neva working in the emergency room, and how she used humor to break the ice and build a rapport with a man that was in obvious pain and was feeling uneasy about his situation.

Neva's Laughter

An aging gentleman walked into the emergency room triage. His hair was matted and blood soaked. His shirt was full of holes and rips, and each hole was surrounded by blood that was oozing from wounds that lay beneath. The man reeked with the smell of alcohol, and it was hard to tell if his stagger was from the loss of blood or his obvious drunkenness. The triage nurse took one look at the man, and she knew immediately that he needed some help. She scrambled around the desk and caught him under one arm and led him over to a wheelchair. Once he was seated, she rushed him straight back to a room alerting the doctor along the way. The charge nurse and the doctor followed the wheelchair. Once the trio found an empty room, they immediately began to work on the man by hooking up the cardiac monitor, obtaining vital signs, and starting an IV. During this time, while the nurses were working, the doctor started interviewing the patient. She started with the obvious question, "what happened?"

The man stared blankly at the doctor for a while not knowing whether or not to answer. He had a look of confusion and concern about him that was a bit unnerving. He shifted around in the bed for a minute, grimacing in pain with each movement. Then, he looked around the room. It appeared that he was sizing up everybody in there before he decided to speak. Then, in a booming slur of words he spoke, "Well hells bells, I guess I had a close encounter with a she-beast. She was a fighter, and thank God she wore out before she killed me."

The doctor stopped in shock. She was puzzled by the man's answer, and she didn't know how to respond. "I don't understand," the doctor replied. "Can you tell me exactly what happened?"

"Why should I?" the man bellowed. "Just sew me up so I can get out of here."

The doctor tensed up a bit due to the patient's abruptness. "I need to know so I can help you," she blurted.

As if solving the mystery in the board game Clue, the man replied, "It was my wife in the kitchen with a meat knife. Now get that bug out of your butt and commence to sewing."

The doctor gave up on the conversation after that, and once his shirt was off the doctor began inspecting the multiple lacerations inflicted by the patient's wife. After some poking and prodding, the doctor said, "these are mostly superficial. I'll be able to close these here," and she turned and left the room.

The man was getting agitated and Neva, the nurse assigned to that room, quickly picked up on the vibe. "What's her problem?" the man asked directing his question to Neva. She didn't know what to say to that comment. So, she decided to change the subject.

"We need to get these wounds cleaned up," she said. The man sat silently while Neva began cleaning the dried blood from his skin. Neva could tell the man was a bit agitated and could feel his anxiety growing. The tension continued getting stronger in the room as she worked. Neva decided to try and talk to the man in an effort to ward off some of his anxiety. She could tell that he was really in pain as he grimaced with each wipe as she scrubbed at the blood.

"I guess you were late for dinner?" Neva said with a smile.

The man sat for a second deep in thought staring at her with cold dark eyes, and then offered a reply, "Yeah and I drank all her wine on the way home." He snickered a bit at this comment. Neva got tickled and let out some laughter. The man's tension eased a bit and he began to relax.

Behind his blood shot eyes and despite the odor of adult beverages on his breath, his jovial spirit and some light-hearted comments came a little more often. Neva and the man continued on talking throughout the suturing process that was being executed by the doctor. After 342 sutures, the doctor quit counting. Neva and the patient continued to tell jokes, and they shared laughter even as she dressed his wounds.

Neva questioned the patient about his medical and social history for the records. Neva found his honesty impressive. The man admitted to drinking at least 12-18 beers a day, indulging in street drugs, and staying out too late for his wife's liking. The man talked candidly about his time in the military and the nightmares of his combat duty.

Neva began to feel a connection with the man as she found out more about him. The man must have felt the same because at one point he reached over and placed his hand on top of Neva's hand and said, "Thanks for your help sweetie. It's nice to know somebody cares."

Neva smiled and continued asking him questions while she was finishing his discharge papers. When it came time for the final question, Neva asked, "When was the last time you had a tetanus shot?" His puzzled look indicated to Neva that he was in need of some further explanation. So, she expanded on the previous question with some more questions: "have you been to the ER in the last 5 years? Stepped on a nail? Had Surgery?"

Through his toothless smile he asked, "I think my wife shot me three years ago. Do you think I got one then?"

Not knowing how to answer, Neva just laughed and shook her head.

Summary

Of course not all patient encounters will be this easy, and there is a time and place for nurses to be serious. Those opportunities present themselves with every turn, but it may not happen often that an opportunity poses itself when a nurse can make an appropriate joke and bring a smile to the patient's face. So, don't let the seriousness of the job interfere with building trust with the patient. Take the time to laugh when appropriate. Be gracious when accepting praise, and reply with a smile. Some people claim that smiles are contagious, and no matter how serious the patient's condition is at that moment the nurse should always remember that the person lying in the bed is a human being and deserving of trust and compassion.

-9-

Treat the Patient, Not the Monitor

"Constant attention by a good nurse may be just as important as a major operation by a surgeon."

-Dag Hammarskjold

Introduction

The field of nursing has come a long way in the past several hundred years. As little as thirty years ago a nurse was required to wear white uniforms and the majority of them were female. Today, nurses are accustomed to wearing scrubs that come in just about every color and style one can think of. The white patent leather shoe has given way to tennis shoes and Crocs. No longer are nurses required to wear a hat; when they are, the hat is usually a surgical cap instead of the little white sailboats.

At one point bedpans were reusable and made of metal versus the plastic disposable bedpans of today. Intravenous fluids came in glass bottles and the tubing that delivered the fluids to patients was made of rubber. Sphygmomanometers were manual and filled with mercury just like the glass thermometers that were in use at the time.

Today, just about everything that touches a patient is disposable and is made of some form of plastic. Today's nurse has the luxury of electronic blood pressure cuffs, SpO2 monitors, and thermometers all-in-one sitting atop rolling carts. The aforementioned items are not the only things in the field of healthcare that has progressed due to the ever-changing technology and the endless studies that have advanced medicine into the twenty-first century.

Technology

Technology is inevitable in the field of medicine, and the technology is a big part of patient care. Nurses must learn to utilize technology as a part of their jobs. Technology changes on a near daily basis, and if a nurse wishes to stay abreast of the latest and greatest patient care tools, then they must actively embrace the changes and be willing to learn new procedures and protocols.

Technology is a must in modern medicine. However, nurses must understand that technology is a tool and not the end-all-be-all in patient care. Nurses must learn to use technology in order to provide better patient care, and not rely on it to step in and replace common sense and good judgment.

The following story illustrates making decisions based on technology rather than an informed and well thought out assessment.

A True Story

There was a female patient that was in an Intensive Care Unit after an extensive twelve-hour surgery. The patient remained intubated after the surgery as a precaution while the anesthesia wore off. After a period of time, the female was extubated. The patient wasn't able to maintain her oxygen saturations, and the patient had to be re-intubated. Keeping the patient sedated was problematic as she kept having break-through episodes where the sedation wasn't working. Several different medications were tried before the doctors were able to find a medication that was effective in keeping the patient sedated.

The husband was witness to everything that the patient was going through. Several days later the patient's blood gases stabilized in the normal range and during rounds on the fifth day the decision was made to wean the patient off the ventilator. The doctors had been sharing all of the information they had concerning the patient's status with her husband all along. The husband had been with the patient the entire time at this point. He was a well-informed spouse and knew as much about his wife's medical history as anyone else did.

The next day, the decision was made to extubate the patient and the procedure was executed without any complications. After doing so, the patient was able to maintain stable readings for an entire day. The patient became coherent and was able to have reasonable conversations with her husband, and she was able to communicate rationally with the doctors and nurses.

However, the second day offered another story. The patient began to desaturate in regards to her oxygen levels. The PCO2 levels were steadily climbing due to the poor oxygen exchange in her lungs secondary to fluid build-up. The doctor had extensive discussions with the husband and gave him instructions on what to look for because the decision was looming about whether or not to re-intubate the patient.

The husband completely understood what signs and symptoms to look for, and he sat patiently bedside waiting and watching for any changes in his wife's condition. The patients PCO2 levels were creeping up, and the patient's mental status was on the decline. She became confused and began talking nonsense and trying to get out of the bed. During each episode her oxygen levels would drop and her heart rate would go up. Her husband was able to calm her and she would immediately fall asleep after being calmed down. While sleeping her heart rate would decrease back within normal limits, and her oxygen saturation would increase back into the normal range. These episodes continued repeatedly and they began happening closer and closer together.

Sometime later, the patient woke up and was having delusions. She was terribly incoherent and her vital signs destabilized as her heart rate climbed into the 120's, and her SpO2 declined into the low 80's. The husband became frantic and stepped outside to find the nurse. As luck would have it, the nurse that was assigned to the patient had to escort her other critical patient down to radiology for a CT scan.

The husband asked the first nurse that walked by if she would come in and check on his wife. During the time period that the husband had been searching for a nurse the patient had fallen back asleep and her vital signs had stabilized. The nurse poked her head into the room, looked right at the monitor, saw that the monitor was not indicating anything out of the normal range, turned to the husband and in a condescending tone said, "Everything is ok. There is nothing wrong here." Without hesitation, the nurse turned and left the scene. The husband was dumbfounded by the nurse's actions and tone. The nurse did not listen to the husband and ignored his concerns in what was deemed as "an over-reacting family member."

After a few minutes, the episode repeated itself. This time the patient was even more irrational and confused as her SpO2 bottomed out at 79%. The husband raced back out of the room and coincidentally the same nurse as before was standing there at the nurses' desk. The husband asked her if she could get the doctor. She began to question the husband and from her tone the husband sensed that the nurse did not care for his opinions. He felt as if the nurse was treating him as some over-reacting frantic person that did not know what he was talking about.

Somewhere in the exchange the nurse made the statement to the husband, "I told you everything was alright." The husband became infuriated at the nurse's lack of respect for him and his sense of urgency. All he could think about was how this nurse was not taking his request seriously and how she was wasting valuable time as his wife was lying in the bed and couldn't breathe.

As his voice rose, he demanded that she tell the doctor to come to his wife's room. The husband's screaming got the attention of everyone in earshot and the room went silent as everyone turned and stared at the two of them. She turned nonchalantly facing the row of desks that lined the nurses' station. The doctor was standing at the far end of the station. She called the doctor's name out across the room. She pointed over her shoulder with her thumb, pumping her arm back and forth toward the husband, and said, "This guy says he needs you. I don't know what he wants. I told him everything was fine."

Without hesitation, the doctor raced around the end of the desk and headed down toward the patient's room. The husband turned and followed the doctor into the room. The doctor looked at the patient. She had a wild and confused stare in her eyes and was speaking incoherently and tugging at her wrist restraints.

The doctor immediately recognized what was occurring with the patient and called for the respiratory team to intubate her. The scene quickly became a frenzy of commotion as people began racing around gathering equipment, preparing medications for sedation, and lying the bed flat as they pulled it away from the wall so they could intubate the patient. One of the nurses escorted the husband from the room and explained what was about to happen, and she assured him that someone would come and get him when the procedure was complete and everything was back in order.

After a short period of time, the doctor opened the door and saw the patient's husband sitting there waiting for some news. The doctor explained to the husband that his wife was resting comfortably and was on a ventilator that was breathing for her. He also explained that it would take some time for everything to get back to normal, but as for now, her vital signs were normal. The doctor immediately apologized for the nurse's behavior, and he offered that there was no excuse for her actions. He told the husband that he had already started an investigation and after speaking with several members of the staff that were witnesses to the episode he had no quantifiable reason that could possibly excuse the nurse's actions. He also told the husband that a nurse manager would be by shortly to speak with him about the event.

In the end, the nurse was severely reprimanded and placed on probation for her actions. The findings showed that the nurse had displayed gross negligence by not performing a proper patient assessment and basing her actions on the monitor readings. The fact that everything on the monitor was stable was irrelevant due to the fact that the machine was not and could not diagnose the underlying problem. The husband was told that it was the nurse's job to find the problem, not the machine's job. The husband was also informed that the only reason the hospital was allowing her to keep her job was the fact that this was the first complaint ever registered against her. It was never revealed as to what actions were brought against the nurse due to her attitude, but the husband assumes something must have happened because for the next two weeks in the ICU he never saw that nurse again.

Main Points

In the case mentioned above, the nurse did not take time to listen to the concerns of the patient's family. She based her decision solely on monitor readings instead of taking the time to assess the situation and then addressing the concerns raised by the husband. This was an error made by the nurse, and in the world of medicine lives are at stake. Errors happen; but more often times than not, the errors can be avoided. Take an extra minute and assess the situation and formulate a plan of action based on a thorough assessment versus a quick look at the monitor readings.

Never make snap decisions. A good nurse relies on information and the best source of information is the patient. In the eyes of the patient, the nurse is deemed the expert by the nature of the business, but this does not mean that the nurse cannot ask for help. It is acceptable for a nurse to say that he or she doesn't know the answer. However, it is not acceptable to ignore the question. Don't be afraid to take a minute and analyze the situation prior to jumping to conclusions based on perceived knowledge. The fact of the matter is that no one person knows everything. Adopting the idea that nurses are not experts in every single aspect of nursing will make the job easier. Keeping one's ego in check is essential. This process is easier said than done.

The demands placed on nurses are almost incomprehensible to someone outside the field. When a nurse is consistently bombarded with questions and expected to answer, it is easy for the nurse to take the position of being the expert. The best way to deal with this situation is to constantly remind one's self that he or she is human just like the patients. If a patient has a question or concern or offers advice on a situation there is always an underlying reason. So, before making a rash decision or spouting out an answer, ensure that a total understanding of the situation surrounding the question or concern is achieved. This takes time, and time is a precious commodity in nursing. The pressures that come with the need for expediency can lead one into a situation that doesn't end well.

With all of these things in mind, the best practice is to slow down, think before speaking, and never underestimate anyone. There is always the possibility that the patient or the patient's family may know more about the situation than the nurse does.

If a patient has a concern the nurse should address that concern before moving on. The field of healthcare is referred to as practicing medicine for a reason. Things are not always black and white and every situation does not always fit nicely into a box. The scenarios stated above can attest to that fact.

In the end, it is in the best interest of a nurse to listen to the patient, treat the needs of the patient with diligence, and don't rely solely on one's personal experience to cloud sound judgment. There is no way for a nurse to know everything about everything, and when nurses are faced with situations that don't follow the norms, nurses should take a step back and analyze the situation. Simply remember that things may not always be as they appear. As in the situation mentioned earlier, everything seemed to be normal according to the monitor, but that was not the case in reality. New nurses are cautioned to use technology only in the best interest of the patient, not what is convenient or the easiest.

-10-

Don't Be That Nurse

"It is not how much you do but how much love you put in the doing."

-Mother Theresa

Introduction

As stated before, nursing is a hard job. Over time, the stress of the job can wear a person down just like a river eroding the landscape in search of the path of least resistance. It is easy to fall into the category of the path of least resistance. However, along this path something always gets washed down stream never to be seen again. Don't be the nurse that gets abused by the elements.

Instead, find a way to use the experiences gained over time to be the river rock standing out in the center that is well rounded, grounded, and sound. Make the elements work in your favor to provide a solid surface that isn't abrasive. Become a rock that others can find refuge on in times of turbulence.

The following ideas can help a nurse smooth off some of the rough edges while avoiding the erosion of one's character, morals, and care.

Passion

If there had to be one word—and only one word—to sum up nursing that word would be "passion." Passion is what drives nurses to get through the day and to deliver care to the sick and ailing. Passion is what makes a nurse get out of the bed in the morning. Passion is what drives a nurse to care. Passion leads to nurturing.

Nurturing leads to healing, and healing is what patient care is all about.

It isn't very hard to spot the nurse that has lost his or her passion. They stick out. They are the ones that complain about everything and spend more time griping about the work that needs to be done rather than actually doing the work. Those people are the nurses that have an excuse for everything and are always trying to pawn work off onto someone else. People scatter when they see those types of nurses coming their direction.

More likely than not, if a person has spent any significant amount of time in a hospital setting, the nurse that is being referred to has been spotted; the crotchety one with a chip on his or her shoulder. The nurse that makes an appearance in a patient's room making the patient feel awkward and uncomfortable. The nurse that has lost passion brings on a sense of impending doom and gloom.

These types of nurses are counterproductive to the goals of healthcare. Nurses are supposed to provide care for the patients in a nurturing fashion. They are not supposed to make the patients feel anxiety or dread. Nurses are supposed to provide care in the pursuit of healing. Mental stress can be just as debilitating as disease. Be a stress reliever instead of a stress giver.

With this in mind, how does one address these issues? First, don't be a problem and there won't be a problem. Being proactive is a must in nursing in every situation, encounter, and process. If you can avoid a problem then do it. Stop the problem before it starts. Mastering the practice of stopping a problem before it starts will lead to a long, happy, and productive career.

One best practice is to be aware. Awareness is mandatory. Be aware of everything. At first this type of awareness might be foreign to a new nurse, but in time, if a nurse works at it this skill will develop. Nursing is all about attention to the details. If the details escape the nurse's attention then bad things can happen.

As with any goal, there has to be an end in sight. A vision must be formulated and one must picture the outcome. If a person envisions himself or herself as the best nurse that has ever existed, and then takes the appropriate steps to reach that goal, he or she can become a great nurse. In order to do this, one must strive to make that vision a reality.

Hardly anyone begins a career of nursing thinking that they will eventually turn into a patient's worst nightmare when he or she loses passion, but it can happen if the appropriate steps are not taken to avoid this pitfall. A conscious decision must be made every day to be the best that they can be and hold on to that vision throughout the entire shift. This takes hard work and a tremendous amount of dedication, but it can be accomplished. Keep the passion for nursing alive, and don't let anyone or anything erode that quality.

Honesty

Another quality that will aid in the prevention of erosion is honesty. Honesty truly is the best policy, and it should be embraced and executed on a daily basis. Be honest with patients, families, doctors, and coworkers and respect will follow. This is another way to be successful as a nurse. No one can tell a new nurse everything to avoid or everything to do to assure that he or she will be viewed as successful, but here are some universal tips that can help.

First, don't make excuses. Florence Nightengale said it best, ""I attribute my success to this - I never gave or took any excuse." Assume the responsibility of good patient care and do everything possible to ensure that the actions necessary to complete patient care are followed through on to the very best of one's ability. Think of it like this, every time a nurse speaks, the words that flow from his or her mouth is a promise. As far as a patient is concerned, the words uttered by a nurse are a solemn oath. Even the simplest words are considered to be a verbal contract written in stone. If a nurse says, "I will be right back," and for whatever reason they do not come right back then the trust has been broken.

Again, honesty truly is the best policy. If a nurse holds true to being honest, the job and the lives of patients will be easier to manage. If a nurse breaks the oath, then the label of being a liar will follow. Once the label has been placed—that nurse lied to me—that label hardly ever gets pulled off. It sticks like super glue, and that is one label that will haunt a nurse throughout the rest of that patient encounter. Think about what is about to be said before making a statement. Instead of saying, "I will be right back," try saying, " I will try to be right back." By adding those two little words—try to—it leaves the nurse an out if something happens that interferes with completing the task in a certain time frame. This way a promise has not been broken if it takes longer than expected to get back to the patient.

One of the best things that a nurse can do is to say what you mean and do what you say. Be honest. No one likes to be lied to even in the best of circumstances, and let's face it, to be sick and to be lied to never makes for a pleasant experience.

Respect

Respect is another key aspect of nursing, and in order to get respect one must earn it. In order to earn respect one must give it. Respect is a two-way street. In the beginning, new nurses will face many challenges revolving around gaining respect. If a patient detects the slightest hesitance from the nurse, the patient will think that the nurse doesn't know what he or she is doing. When this happens, patient care becomes harder for the nurse, and the patient won't respond well to the care if the patient doesn't respect the nurse's abilities. In order to avoid this problem, the nurse must be confident and display polished behaviors at all times. No one has ever stated that being a nurse is easy, at least not in earnest. Nurses are under the microscope—so to speak—every minute of every shift and sometimes even beyond that.

One way to earn respect from the patient is to keep the patient informed. Tell the patient everything that is going on. Never, never, never walk into a patient's room and just start giving medicines or start a procedure. If a nurse barges in and starts stabbing the patient without warning, then the patient automatically starts the disliking process. By sharing information, the nurse slowly earns the respect of the patient because the nurse is now treating the patient as an equal. If a nurse just starts doing procedures without explaining the procedure to the patient, the patient can view the nurse as rude or worse. The patient will interpret these actions as being condescending. The patient may think that the nurse either doesn't care or that the patient cannot comprehend what is happening. Neither of those scenarios will gain the nurse any respect from the patient.

Aside from the patients, new nurses must gain respect from their coworkers. The easiest way to do this is to be a good listener. As far as seasoned nurses are concerned, new nurses don't know anything. Therefore, the new nurse is expected to listen and learn. It will take some time and effort to remove the stigma of ignorance. In reality, a new nurse may be very good and very effective in the job, but as far as the other nurses are concerned a new nurse is ignorant. It will take a while for a new nurse to break free from this stereotype, and in the beginning it is best for a new nurse to understand that his or her opinion may be viewed the same way that people view the opinion of a child— with little regard.

As far as some nurses are concerned, they don't want the new person's opinion because it has not yet earned any merit. Also, there is the possibility that one's opinion and or actions will never earn any merit with some nurses. Some nurses will never treat a new nurse as an equal because they have more experience than the new person. Therefore the new guy will always be viewed as less credible to the seasoned veteran. Don't be disheartened when this happens. Not all nurses are this way, but among the ones that are, they always get the most attention because those types of nurses are the ones that are easy to remember.

Furthermore, one should not be alarmed if certain other nurses never give any respect to a new nurse. Some nurses are just callous in this aspect and don't like anybody that is not familiar to them. This harsh fact is just the way that some nurses behave. The correctness of these ideas is not in consideration at this point, but it is best to understand that these types of actions do in fact happen. In essence, a new nurse should not be surprised if a certain amount of hazing occurs. However, it is best to learn to avoid the nitpickers when possible and avoid the pitfalls of becoming one of those nurses by joining in on the bad behavior.

Treat your co-workers with the same amount of respect that you expect from them. The worse thing a new nurse can do is to develop a superiority complex. This kind of behavior can become self-destructive. Think of co-workers as part of a team rather than a competition. Don't get caught up trying to one-up another co-worker. Nobody likes a know-it-all.

More likely than not, every person in the healthcare field will run across a nurse that is a self-proclaimed genius during his or her career, and in some instances there can be many of them at one time. This is where it can get dangerous for a new and impressionable nurse. Avoid the temptation of becoming one of those nurses. Surround yourself with the nurses that enjoy their jobs and want to be there. Stay away from the complainers and soon you will earn the respect of everyone around you.

Remember that actions speak louder than words, and remember that body language is the first language that a person learns, even before learning to speak. If a person displays an air of confidence rather than an air of condescension, he or she will be accepted as a person of integrity quicker than others.

The following statement holds true for all nurses. If a nurse wishes to make friends and get help—when needed—don't look down one's nose at co-workers. Treat every co-worker as an equal. This is especially true when it comes to techs, nurse's aides, LPNs, and janitorial staff. Think about it. These people can be very helpful in a pinch, or they can make the nurse's job a miserable one. If a nurse treats co-workers poorly, most likely the co-workers will do the same thing back to the nurse. Even though others may not be as highly trained as a Registered

Nurse, they are in-and-out of the patients' rooms as much as anybody else. These people can be a nurse's first line of defense in avoiding problems or alerting the nurse when things aren't going exactly as planned.

For instance, if the custodian notices that a patient is having problems breathing and alerts the nurse to the situation it makes the nurse look good. If the custodian chooses not to speak up because he or she believes that the nurse will not listen to them, then the nurse has failed because the patient is ultimately the nurse's responsibility. The liability doesn't rest on the custodian's shoulders, but it does rest on the nurse's.

Also, give some respect to paramedics. Even though they don't necessarily work in the hospital or for the hospital, they do take responsibility for the patient during transports. They are trained professionals and should be treated as such. Paramedics work under a different set of rules than nurses do, and this can create some problems due to the misunderstandings of one another's jobs. However, ignorance does not excuse bad behavior from either party. The ability to listen and learn can go a long way in gaining and earning respect.

Doctors are another story. They have the ultimate say when it comes to patient care. With this in mind it is best to tread lightly when there is a difference of opinion between doctors and nurses. Doctors give orders for a reason, and if the order is not followed to the letter, then nothing good can come from it. It is a nurse's job to follow the doctor's orders. However, this does not mean that nurses are not allowed to question the doctor's order if the nurse does not understand the order. But before questioning the doctor it is best to have a well thought out plan containing thoughtful questions and reasoning behind the questions before approaching the doctor. Doctors by nature don't mind teaching nurses, but they don't appreciate being undermined or questioned openly or publicly. Use the utmost tact and discretion when questioning the doctor. Don't be a bull in a china shop because this can earn a nurse a bad reputation. Don't be intimidated or afraid to speak up, but use common courtesy when doing so.

Caring

Being a nurse is all about caring. Care for the best interest of the patients, care about the job, and taking care of oneself will lead a nurse to a long and successful career. By following these three simple rules a nurse can make a difference.

Saying these things is easy, but following through on the ideas is another. The best way to maintain a positive attitude is to avoid the grumps. Don't get caught up in the griping and complaining. Every nurse has a reason to complain because the job is hard and there are always extenuating circumstances that can make a nurse miserable. But, instead of dwelling on the negatives look for the positives. By doing so, a nurse will stay true to the task at hand, and this allows a nurse to avoid the temptation of letting emotion override logic. It is easy to be a complainer, and it is hard to stay dedicated due to the fatigue and the stresses of the job. However, there is one thing that will always carry a nurse through the daily grind, which is the fact that if a nurse does the job and does it well, the nurse will make a difference in someone's life.

Be the nurse that everyone enjoys being around versus the nurse that people go run and hide from. Be the nurse that has a positive impact on the people around them, but don't be the nurse that exudes negative energy. Be the nurse that cares, instead of the nurse that is simply drawing a paycheck. Be caring, and don't be condescending. Be the best by showing a willingness to learn, and work hard all day— every day. Don't be the nurse that tries to use convenience as a crutch rather than to go the extra mile. Don't avoid the work; instead, embrace it like you would a child. Hold the work dear to your heart, and don't fall into a rut that leads to burn out.

Caring has many faces and each patient will be different in needs and wants. Some patients are independent and may only want a little support while other patients can be very demanding and want everything done for them. Be careful not to stereotype patients too quickly as this can lead to misjudgment. It is impossible to foresee every possible scenario that can play out in a patient encounter. It is best to be open and listen to the needs of the patient and then decide on the best plan of action. Being attentive and honest is always a good policy. Don't make promises that you cannot or will not keep. Don't judge patients by their beliefs and support structure. Be the nurse that cares and wants to help the patient in his or time of need. If it takes an extra minute to figure out what the patient really wants and or needs, then give the extra minute. Even if rushed, don't act like it. Always make the patient that is in front of you the focus of your attention. If distracted the patient will know, and patients perceive distraction as not caring because the focus is somewhere else instead of on the patient where it should be.

Never discount a patient's intuitiveness. Don't fall prey to the urge to think that the title of nurse makes a person smarter than the patient. Remember that nurses are people also. Nurses can get sick just like anyone else, and there is a possibility that the patient in your care is a nurse and hasn't told you that fact. Always expect the unexpected.

Be kind, be happy, be caring, be respectful, be willing, be ready, be honest, and everything else will fall into place. The best advice ever given when it comes to nursing is to always follow the golden rule: do unto others, as you would have others do unto you.

About the Authors

Lance Hansard has 20 years experience in the field of Emergency Medicine and has a Master's Degree in Professional Writing from Kennesaw State University.

Richard Lamphier is a 30-year veteran of nursing who is currently working for the biggest children's healthcare system in Georgia. Richard holds numerous Instructor certifications and has had a vast and exciting career as a nurse while working in burn units, Mobile Intensive Care Units, air transports for critically ill patients, and as an education consultant.

Working together on Mobile Intensive Care Units and air ambulances, Lance and Richard decided to put their experience and talents together to write the book, *Registered Nursing: Tips & Tidbits.*